Hot Summer Nights

Hot Summer Nights

A Month in the ER

Dr. S

Writers Club Press
San Jose New York Lincoln Shanghai

Hot Summer Nights
A Month in the ER

Writers Club Press
an imprint of iUniverse.com, Inc.

For information address:
iUniverse.com, Inc.
5220 S 16th, Ste. 200
Lincoln, NE 68512
www.iuniverse.com
See also:
www.dr-s-md.com

ISBN: 0-595-16924-4

Printed in the United States of America

This book is dedicated to my family.

Contents

Acknowledgements

I especially want to thank the many health care professionals, and all the others that have contributed to the unique experience that is my life.

Introduction
"Sipping at the fire hydrant..."

With all the ER programs on television these days there is a real focus on the dramatic in medicine. It occurred to me that some folks might be interested in what the practice of Emergency Medicine is really like in the vast majority of hospitals around the country.

Unlike on television, the majority of Emergency Department cases are things that would normally be treated in a doctor's office, but for whatever reason, the patient presents to the Emergency Room. Federal law requires that they are all seen, evaluated, and provided appropriate stabilizing treatment. This is all of part of federal governmental regulation known as EMTALA (the Emergency Medical Treatment and Active Labor Act).

More than anything else, Emergency Medicine can be best described as long hours of boredom and frustration punctuated by minutes of sheer panic. Popular media tends to compress all the crazy moments into a single nugget of content. In reality, they are randomly interspersed throughout any given day.

Another observation that I have made is that there are many misconceptions about the role and capabilities of an Emergency Department. Our real job is to identify and address life-threatening conditions, and the tools we have are biased towards that end. Our job is not to necessarily figure out what is wrong with a patient. Most of the time we are able to do this, but it is not really our charter; that is the job of the primary care physician. Patients frequently confuse our role with that of the primary care physician, and seek care in the Emergency Department because they think we are better equipped to figure out their medical problem. This frequently leads to a very expensive medical investigation; we are obligated to rule out improbable life-threatening conditions rather than focus on a probable diagnosis.

It occurred to me that perhaps the best way to give folks a real flavor of what is involved in the practice of Emergency Medicine is to capture the essence of what I see in a given month of shift work in a small city Emergency Department. I felt that this was a more accurate reflection of emergency medicine in general; the bulk of Emergency Room visits across the country occurs in this type of facility rather than at a large regional trauma center. I had worked at both types of facilities and had found that their patient cross sections were similar with an important difference. Regional facilities act as referral centers and get clusters of cases that cannot be handled in smaller facilities. This is usually due to the lack of some specific local resource, such as a neurosurgical consultant, or in-house cardiac catheterization capability. Regional centers also don't see very common medical issues strictly because they are addressed by referring hospitals. An example of this is appendicitis. It's a fairly common affliction, but rarely makes it to the regional hospital.

The small city Emergency Department sees it all. They are typically the only facility in the city, and they usually provide medical care for a broad expanse of the surrounding rural area as well. This "catchment area" is often two or more times the size of the city the hospital serves.

Something else that needs some introduction is the structure and operation of an Emergency Department. These are really team affairs. When an Emergency Department is working well it is very much like a symphony. The emergency physician is the conductor who coordinates the activity of all the players. The nurses and technicians see to the activities within the department. The ancillary services (laboratory, radiology, respiratory, etc) provide services on demand. Local primary care physician and Consultants are both a resource and a point of pass-off for many cases. Police, Fire Department, Ambulance Services, and the like are our proxy with the community. All of this has to work together smoothly for an Emergency Department to be effective.

As I have already stated, my goal in this book is to introduce as much realism as I can to a snapshot of the practice of emergency medicine. This may offend some folks, but that is a risk of the writing business. Though I may make some derogatory comments and the like, it is not that I bear any ill will towards others; it is usually because of the frustration of the moment. Similarly, there is a segment of the medical community that has a vested interest in maintaining an altruistic and idealistic perception of medicine among the public. To them I apologize in advance, and suggest they find another book to read.

Emergency Medicine is about medical cases, and so most of this book addresses cases. The vast majority of these cases are really very generic, and I cover them in that manner. Any information that would betray confidentiality is omitted. The reality is that such information would not really be germane to this book anyway. I attempt to capture the cases, their flow through the Emergency Department, the thought that goes into investigating them, the medical issues involved, and the final disposition. You will find that I often expound on the frustrations we face. These are real issues common to most facilities, and can provide interesting insights into the Emergency Department and their patients.

Finally, it is worth noting that this is a cross section through a month in the Emergency Department. I have arbitrarily chosen a month in the summer because this is when I had the free time to do this project. As you might imagine, this does bias the cases to what you see in the summer. An interesting follow-up might be a month in the winter. If there is enough interest, I will write a wintertime sequel to this book.

Shift 1
"Boredom is a good thing..."

Wednesday—24 Hours

Noon

It's another hot and humid summer day. On arrival, the slate is clear, at least for now. The nature of Emergency Medicine is fickle though, and the department can be completely full five minutes from now.

Before I leap into the fray, it might be helpful to generally describe the department. We are a full service Emergency Department that sees roughly 14,000 patients a year. The city has a population of roughly 30,000, and we have a catchment area of perhaps three times that. In the department we have two urgent care rooms, three general-purpose rooms, a two bay trauma room, an outpatient surgery room, and a cardiac room. If necessary, we can recruit two additional urgent care rooms, plus the entire outpatient area of roughly six bays. We mix and match the rooms to meet the demand. Well, on with it...

There is time to chat with the nurses for a while; we usually have three nurses and one administrative technician in the department. The topic of the day is stocks, and what our latest favorite is likely to be doing. This doesn't last long as patients start rolling in.

My first case of the day is a 39-year-old white male with upper abdominal pain for months, worse since this morning. It is sharp, mid-abdominal, and radiates to his back. He's had similar episodes in the past, but this is the worst. He's never had this investigated in the past.

This is a real road-warrior kind of guy, with poor hygiene and filthy cloths. Surprisingly, prior to arrival, he had actually called a doctor he had seen in the past. He was to be seen in the office in about an hour, but of course instead he presented to my Emergency Room.

When we get to the part of our interview where I ask about alcohol intake, he's rather put off. "I'm not an alcoholic," he says. Apparently, his nurse had already covered this ground. I try and defuse the defensiveness by explaining why we have to ask the question; that it can help us determine those things he is most at risk for that can cause abdominal pain. I finally get, "I only have 6-12 beers a day."

The exam is unremarkable except for an enlarged liver and mid-epigastric (middle upper abdomen) tenderness. He's shaky and hypertensive, consistent with alcoholic withdrawal. I start our routine abdominal pain work-up. This includes blood-work, a urinalysis, and abdominal X-rays. My suspicion is acute pancreatitis (an inflammation of the pancreas common in alcoholics). However, it could just as easily be half a dozen other things. This is why I do pretty much the same work-up for everyone with abdominal pain (adjusted for age and sex related differences). We'll see.

Meanwhile I see a 17-year-old white male in no obvious distress. He complains of 5 days of headache, body aches, and a sore throat. He hasn't bothered to contact his regular doctor, but comes to my Emergency Room instead; do you begin to see a pattern here? His exam is normal. His lab is normal; he doesn't have a strep infection (Streptococci pyogenes, the most common bacterial cause of a sore throat).

Then I get the real kicker, the real agenda, "Oh, by the way, I really can't go to work with this. I need a note for a couple days off."

This is a point where hospital politics comes into play. The directive from hospital administration is to maximize customer service and minimize complaints. Somehow over the last several years, medicine has changed to what I call "McMedicine." Hospital administration pressures the Emergency Department to give the patient what they want in order to minimize complaints. Of course, they also want us to minimize expenses and maximize revenues. This has obvious potential for a range of Catch-22s.

This guy may have a viral syndrome; he is definitely demonstrating some medical malingering. Let's keep everybody happy. I gave him his get-out-of-jail-free card. He can take some Tylenol or Motrin like the rest of us.

Back to our 39-year-old road warrior. Bingo, his pancreatic enzymes are elevated. Looks like he's working on the acute pancreatitis that I suspected. This is a disorder that can produce severe pain, and can have a range of life threatening complications. I get him admitted quickly and out of my hair.

Next is a 3-year-old white female with a 4-5 day history of painful urination. I had seen her several days ago with a normal exam and normal urinalysis. She was later seen by her regular doctor, and started on Suprax (an antibiotic that would even work well for a urinary tract infection) for an ear infection. Allegedly, she was having increased pain with urination, and "she has only urinated twice in the last three days!" She was scheduled to see regular doctor later this afternoon, but instead presented to my Emergency Room. I have to bite my tongue.

This patient did have some urethral irritation, but is otherwise normal. I start her on some Lotrisone (a topical antifungal-steroid combination). She can follow-up with her regular doctor.

Two squads hit our door at about the same time. They are both direct admissions to the hospital. They are whisked through our department and up to the floor. Yesss!

We are so frequently the dumping-ground for local physician's problem patients. It is so good when they actually take responsibility for them.

It's down time again. Given that it's mid-afternoon mid-week it should be relatively quiet till the local doctor's offices close at 5:00 PM.

This might be an appropriate point to bring up Emergency Room lore. I use the term "Quiet" with some caution. Emergency Department workers are a very superstitious lot. "Quiet" is considered the "Q"-word. We (half-seriously) feel that using the word can jinx us with a lot of work. There are a lot of words we don't use much. Another that comes to mind is the word, "Slow". You can make the association as to why we don't like that term.

Something else we often discuss among ourselves is how things come in threes. This seems surprisingly true: three chest pains, three lacerations, three pelvic pains, etc. Life is so strange.

We also frequently discuss our "Karma" or our "Black Clouds." It really does sometimes seem that when certain of us work together we routinely have miserably chaotic shifts. Now it may just be the time of day and week we're are working, it's hard to say.

Oops. Trauma time. The scanner has Life-Flight on standby. A pickup truck seems to have been struck by a fully loaded semi tractor-trailer. This is a situation of a very movable object, and an irresistible force. It sounds like no one won, and squads are inbound.

Okay. The first victim is a 49-year-old white male. He was an unrestrained passenger in the semi. Looking at the picture that the fire department brought with them, the semi didn't fare very well either. He was apparently knocked unconscious, as he has no recollection of the accident. His primary complaint is right facial and right arm pain. He has lots of road rash. He's wearing a cervical collar and is on a backboard. We'll get multiple films and a scan of his head and see what all we've got.

Meanwhile I see the 47-year-old while male driver of the pickup. He too was unrestrained. His truck was creamed, but he seems to have come out of it with minimal injuries. He complains of right face, left elbow, and left knee pain. He too was brought in with a cervical collar and on a backboard. He'll get a lot of films here as well.

The driver of the semi refused rescue squad transport to the Emergency Room for evaluation.

While the traumas are off to the X-ray department, I take time to see a 39-year-old white male who was sent over from one of the local manufacturing companies. He cut his elbow on a piece of metal at work. It's a simple laceration with no complications. Six sutures and, bam, on the road again.

Okay, back to the trauma. The pickup driver managed a broken nose multiple cuts and abrasion. The semi passenger wound up with a concussion, and lots of abrasions. They were both pretty lucky. We discharged them with follow-up as appropriate.

Surprise, surprise, we've just been informed that the driver of the semi is on the way in. Seems that as time has passed he's feeling more uncomfortable. We'll see if he shows up...

We're back to having a few minutes of down time. The nurses and tech are harassing me.

Here's a winner. A 19-month-old white female was put on the hood of the car while her mother took in the groceries. Ha, wouldn't you know it, the child fell off onto her head. There was no loss of consciousness thankfully, and the child has been doing fine since. Cervical spine X-rays are done and normal. This complements a normal exam. Prior to discharge, her mother wants a prescription for Tylenol so that Medicaid will pay for it. Here is our tax dollars at work.

Oh joy, oh joy, a 37-year-old white female with a "migraine headache" for 5 days. This is just like her prior headaches. It's just not getting better, and she wants a shot for it. Of course she hasn't taken anything for this headache, and couldn't be bothered to contact her regular doctor.

A real problem in Emergency Rooms is drug seekers. These are folks with concocted stories trying to con the doctors into giving them prescription pain medicines. Unfortunately, pain is not something that can be quantitatively assessed, and so it can be difficult to ferret these folks out. They usually come in complaining of headache, back pain, tooth pain, or belly pain. They are also typically "allergic" to every pain medicine except their drug of choice.

Some folks will take the drug-seeking act to the point of allowing procedures to be done on them, as long as they get the pain medicine they are looking for. I've personally had folks take the charade to the point of allowing a lumbar puncture. It really has you scratching your head.

We as physicians are criticized for not adequately treating pain. Then we're told in the same breath that prescription pain medicine abuse is rising to all-time levels. Go figure…

This patient accepts what I give her and goes away. As long as they don't demand a scheduled drug like Demerol or morphine (both are narcotic pain medicines), I usually give them what they want. Again, this is McMedicine, drive through service with a smile. It cuts down on complaints and keeps administration off our back.

Luckily the Emergency Physicians at this facility are consistent when it comes to narcotics and headaches. This hasn't always been the case. When we had docs that gave narcotics in a cavalier fashion, hardly a shift would go by that you wouldn't have a half dozen patients come in demanding them, usually Demerol. Then, if you'd actually cave on the issue and give them what they wanted, you invariably see another half dozen patients swoop in with the same request. Since we've consistently stopped this practice, we've dramatically reduced the numbers of drug seekers. And most of the remaining patients that keep coming in will accept non-narcotic options and go away.

6:00 PM

It's evening time and things are heating up. The doctors offices are closed, and now every little ache and pain is a crisis.

I've got a 15-year-old white male with a legitimate complaint. He was at football practice and injured his right small finger. We film it. Nothing's broken, but he did manage to dislocate it. A little traction and it pops right back where it belongs. He is splinted and out the door.

The next gentleman, and I use that term loosely, is a 25-year-old white male who states he has had a fever, sore throat, nausea and diarrhea for a week. He usually sees doctor NONE. His exam is benign, except for all of the body and tongue piercings. His lab is normal. It all sounds like a viral syndrome. But, wouldn't you know it, he wants off from work for a few days…"You deserve a break today, so get up and get away to…" Service with a smile.

I love my job. I love my job.

Now for a 5-year-old white male with a two hour history of low grade fever and sore throat. Can you believe this? He had just finished a course of Zithromax (an antibiotic with good coverage for Strep), but his mother is still sure he has strep throat. Guess what? Not. He does have a couple of oral ulcers and the start of a faint red rash on his hands. He probably has hand foot and mouth disease. This is a viral infection (Coxsackie A virus) that causes a fever and sore throat. We've seen a lot of it over the past month, and guess what? It requires only symptomatic treatment.

Then we have a 54-year-old obese white female with three weeks of right hip pain. She comes in tonight because, "I've been putting up with this for three weeks now. Then I said to myself, 'I have insurance, I'm tired of dealing with this, so I'm going to have this looked at right now.'" Of course this patient has a physician that she hasn't bothered to contact any time over the last three weeks, nor has she has tried anything over-the-counter. She has a trochanteric bursitis (inflammation of the bursa over the hip-bone) that would have responded to almost any over-the-counter anti-inflammatory medicines like Motrin or Aleve. Of course, since she is in the Emergency Room, she expects to walk away with a cure. I give her a script for prescription strength Aleve (which is the same as taking two over-the-counter variety).

Well talk about it and it is likely to walk in. I was just talking to the nurses about how much I dislike seeing women with abdominal pain. It invariably requires that I do a pelvic examination that I don't like doing and she doesn't like having done. Here we have a 22-year-old white female with a transient mid-abdominal pain. She has been having unprotected sex and is on no birth control. Of course she is worried that she might be pregnant. She tried a home pregnancy test that was negative, but doesn't trust the test. She is symptom free on presentation. She has a normal exam, and normal lab. And guess what? She's not pregnant. The moral of the story: USE BIRTH CONTROL if you're going to have sex and don't want to risk pregnancy. Further, it seems like no one is using condoms any more. Last time I checked, things like AIDS is still out there, and we have our share of AIDS patients that visit us here. It just seems like folks are living in denial.

Then I see a 10-year-old white male who had stepped on a nail a week ago. He has been on two different antibiotics in the last week. Today he has a grape-sized, red, volcano-like swelling on the top of his foot. I lanced it and gobs of pus rushed out. I cultured it. Pseudomonas (a difficult to treat bacteria) is a possibility with these types of wounds. Hopefully he doesn't get an infection of the bone; that can lead to amputation. I get lab and films to get a better feel for the extent of the infection. We'll see.

Meanwhile a 3-year-old white male ran into the corner of his mom's hutch and lacerated his left cheek. It's a small cut, but not in a good location for Dermabond (a suture-less skin glue). It took three stitches, but he did surprisingly well with it.

Wow. Look out, one of my nurses is on a tear. She doesn't like how a cupboard door is latched, so she whipped out a screwdriver and removed the offending latch—problem solved.

Back to the 10-year-old with the foot lesion. The lab and films are good. He gets a shot of broad spectrum antibiotic and will be seen again in the morning by his regular doctor.

The witching hour is approaching and people are trying to get to bed. If they can't sleep then they often end up in my Emergency Room. In this case it is a 16-month-old white female with fussiness and fever since the morning. Of course it's a crisis now. The child has an ear infection, and is easily fixed. It could have been handled earlier in the day or tomorrow morning. A little Tylenol or Motrin could have gone a long way. Ah well, sometimes I don't know why these things still upset me.

The security guys asked me what I was doing. I'm busily typing into my PDA via a portable keyboard. They tell me if I don't include them in my book they well hunt me down. Well they have now been officially mentioned.

Security, as well as the local police, are entities that are essential to all Emergency Departments. We tend to see all of the unsavory characters that our community has to offer. Many of them, like the despondent overdoses or the hopped up crank-heads, are often brought in kicking, screaming, biting, and the like. It can take six to eight big guys to hold these folks down until they can be adequately restrained. Then we get our share of patient lovelies with knives, guns, and the like. And let's not forget the occasional death threats. It's a lively work-place that makes you look forward to being on the job.

Next is something we see a lot of, an 11-year-old white male with a two hour history of hives. There has been no particular new exposure. These are typically caused by an allergic reaction to something. We rarely identify the offending agent. In this kid, the rash was getting better spontaneously. A little bit of Benadryl (an antihistamine) sped the process along. This is an over-the-counter medicine that could have been given at home.

12:00 AM

So now its midnight and time for the "Real" emergencies. I have a 59-year-old white female who had a bladder suspension a week ago (this corrects a common cause of urinary incontinence in women). She hasn't had a bowel movement since, and now it's a crisis. Code brown, we are about to have a code brown. For this emergency, we use the traditional high hot and hell of a lot (a soap suds enema). Oh what a relief it is…

Now what I would have liked to have said to this patient and patients like this is, "Every grocery store has a magical aisle. On one side is stuff that slows you down, and on the other is stuff that knocks the crap out of you. Take your pick."

The only thing worse than folks coming in on their own with constipation is when the local doctors send them over from their offices because they don't want to deal with it. This is usually without even the courtesy of a call. It would be interesting to know just how many millions of dollars is spent in Emergency Rooms in any given year giving enemas.

Zzzz…

I take every opportunity I get to take a short nap. This is a survival trait I learned in residency. There, depending on your rotation, you might be on continuous duty for as much as 30 days at a time. You develop the ability to sleep any time, anywhere, under any conditions. If you don't, you have a hard time making it through the training program.

2:00 AM and the sleepless begin to arrive. The first case is a 7-month-old white female with a fever and fussiness through the day. She hasn't had Tylenol since yesterday morning. The mother either can't afford more or doesn't want to pay for it, so she brings her child to our facility. Of course the symptoms are no worse now than 18 hours ago, but it's keeping everyone up. The picture is a viral syndrome, there are no localizing signs or symptoms, and the fever defervesces with Tylenol. I give her mother a prescription so Medicaid (you and I) can pay for her Tylenol.

This is followed immediately by a 17-year-old white male with nausea, vomiting, and left-sided abdominal pain for a few hours. However, by the time he presents, his symptoms have fully resolved. So why did he come? Who knows? He wants to be checked. Of course everything's normal. This is likely just another viral bug. He goes home with the recommendation to use symptomatic medicines, and follow-up as needed.

Zzzz…

It's 5 AM and my call to reveille is a 74-year-old white female who had had two episodes of right face and hand tingling lasting for seconds. This patient has metastatic (widely disseminated) breast cancer and is already fully anticoagulated on the blood thinner, Coumadin. Things that immediately come to mind are an intra-cerebral bleed (given the blood thinner), or a metastatic lesion in the brain (given the underlying cancer). I do a range of lab as well as a CT Scan of her head, and everything is as normal as it's going to be for this patient. There isn't a lot to offer.

The goal with these terminal patients is to try and keep them out of the hospital as much as possible. They typically have little time left and it should be spent with their family and such rather than lying around in a hospital. Not to mention their real infection risk given the organisms they would be exposed to in the hospital. They are typically immune compromised and don't need to be around other sick folks. I try to help provide the best quality of life for whatever life these folks have left.

In this case, the patient will go home, and follow up with her regular physician. She wants to go home, so that is a plus. I often weigh their desires, and we sometimes do social admits to give family and patient a rest. This is strictly against the rules of the payers, but it's a fact of life.

6:00 AM

Time for breakfast, SOS (Shit on a Shingle as they called in my military days), yum yum. Not...

Then we have an 87-year-old white male who comes in by squad with 3 days of progressive shortness of breath. He has been under treatment for chronic atrial fibrillation, congestive heart failure, and coronary artery disease. He has also had an angioplasty in the recent past.

Atrial Fibrillation is a heart arrhythmia where the top of the heart acts erratically. The bottom of the heart picks up the erratic electrical activity from above and tries to respond to it. This often leads to a very fast irregular heartbeat where the beats are ineffective in pumping blood. This can lead to a range of symptoms from syncope (passing out), to chest pain, to pulmonary edema. Longer term, it produces turbulent flow in the upper chambers of the heart that can predispose to blood clots. These can break off and lodge in the brain producing a stroke.

There are many approaches to dealing with Atrial Fibrillation depending on how long it has been present, and the symptoms it is causing. The key issues in management are rate control, restoration of a normal rhythm, and reduction of stroke risk. Rate control is typically done with medicines that block the conduction of the erratic upper heart signal from the lower heart. Restoration of a normal rhythm is done either with electrical cardioversion or antiarrhythmics medicines. Stroke risk reduction is done with some form of anticoagulation.

In this patient there is chronic atrial fibrillation. This means that, for whatever reason, his doctors were unable to keep him in a normal rhythm. Because of this, he was on a rate controlling medicine, Lanoxin, and a stroke prevention medicine, Coumadin.

Congestive heart failure is a common, though imprecise term. It usually means that, due to some underlying cardiac pathology, the heart is unable to keep up with the demands placed upon it. In the case of Left Heart failure you wind up with congestion upstream that, in this case means the lungs. Simplistically, you wind up with increased vascular pressures within the lungs, tissue fluids leak through into the alveoli (air sacs) and you end up with pulmonary edema (fluid in the lungs). This can be treated in a couple of ways. You can either try and make the pump work better, or you can reduce the work it needs to do.

Coronary artery disease is the "hardening of the arteries" that is so much talked about. It's essentially a lifetime accumulation of cholesterol plaqueing in the lining of heart vessels that narrow their lumen until there is inadequate blood flow when the heart is under load. This is usually asymptomatic until a critical threshold is reached. When it does become symptomatic, a person typically has angina. Angina is a chest pressure that may radiate into the neck or down the arms; it may also be associated with nausea, sweating, and shortness of breath. Stable angina occurs when a similar amount of exertion reliably reproduces these symptoms. Unstable angina occurs when these symptoms are occurring at rest. Unstable angina is the more worrisome as it may herald an impending heart attack. A heart attack, or acute myocardial infarction, is when a cholesterol plaque ruptures or a small spontaneous clot lodges in a narrowed heart vessel. The symptoms are typically like angina, only they are worse and do not resolve. Coronary artery disease is treated in a number of ways. It may be treated with some combination of medicine, angioplasty, or bypass. Angioplasty is the use of a catheter directed balloon to expand a narrowed heart artery and improve flow. It is worth noting that this is not a permanent fix, and these vessels tend to re-occlude, some sooner than later.

After this long-winded explanation it is easier to have some insight into what might be going on with our 87-year-old patient. He's having progressive shortness of breath without chest pain. His oxygenation is fine, and his chest X-ray does not show heart failure. His EKG shows his chronic atrial fibrillation, but in addition, it shows new ischemic changes on the lateral aspect of his heart. This suggests that that part of the heart is not getting enough blood flow to adequately oxygenate the heart muscle.

This brings up the specter of an exception to the rule. In this patient, his shortness of breath is likely an anginal equivalent. An anginal equivalent is a set of atypical symptoms that still means the heart is not getting enough blood to some area. It is more common in diabetics who have damage to small nerves about the heart, and thus don't transmit the pain signals appropriately. In this patient though, who knows? In reality it is a moot point. He's a keeper. His regular doctor is contacted and he is whisked upstairs for further treatment. He's likely to get another cardiac catheterization before he goes home. I'm betting he's re-occluded one of his vessels.

It seems to be a cardiac morning. Next is a 75-year-old white female with a history of an infiltrative cardiomyopathy (stuff, usually an abnormal protein, within the substance of the heart that doesn't belong there, and that impairs its function). She was just in the hospital with congestive heart failure that had been effectively treated with medicine. She had had a normal heart catheterization two years ago, and a normal DSE (Dobutamine Stress Echo) just two days ago; this makes is unlikely that there is any significant narrowing of her heart arteries.

A Dobutamine Stress Echo is a non-invasive functional heart study that looks for ischemia in a heart under load. It is usually performed on folks that would have a difficult time walking on a treadmill. A medicine that speeds up the heart, dobutamine, is infused through an IV, and cardiac response is monitored by a special kind of ultrasound called an Echocardiogram. Areas of the heart that don't get enough blood flow under load are slowed, hypokinetic. This allows you to pretty much pin-point what heart vessels are narrowed.

This patient has been having chest burning for days that's better with Mylanta, but is concerned that this could be her heart. Her EKG is unchanged, her chest X-ray is baseline, and her lab is normal. Her symptoms are cured with a GI Cocktail (Maalox and Viscous Lidocaine). Though angina can sometimes be improved with a GI Cocktail, it is improbable that she is having anything other than GERD (gastroesophageal reflux or heartburn). You really can't develop significant coronary artery narrowing in just a couple of years (even given her underlying cardiac pathology), and the DSE two days ago provides additional reassurance. She is put on Prilosec (a stomach acid reducing medicine), given reflux instructions (foods to avoid, things to try), and advised to follow-up with her regular doctor.

With so many patients you never really know for sure. Lay people have the misconception that we deal with certainties in medicine. In reality, medical certainty is just an estimation of relative risk for a given patient. From the standpoint of the Emergency Medicine Physician, it is the relative risk he is willing to accept that the patient will not leave the Emergency Department and promptly have a significant medical event. Every doctor has their own threshold. Often it is set by the number of (bad) experiences they have had along the way in patient care; sometimes it is just based on a gut feeling. In this patient, the relative risk is acceptable to me, and the patient is discharged with follow-up. She has real disease that is going to cause her further problems in the future, but it is my estimation that the burning sensation she has been having is not cardiac in origin.

Just a few more comments on gut feelings, or intuition, seems in order at this point. I have lost track of the number of times this has saved me from peril. You might have a patient with a nonspecific complaint, who's had multiple normal studies done recently, and doesn't have any real specific findings on your evaluation. However, you have this nagging suspicion that something significant is going on despite your inability to find out what it might be. Then you usually have to convince the local physician to admit and further evaluate the patient based on your feeling. This in itself can be a daunting task, and sometimes requires heated arguments. You feel vindicated when, minutes or hours later, the patient has a significant event that they likely would not have survived had they been at home.

Well, back to the story. Following on the heels of our last patient is an 87-year-old white female with dizziness, nausea and vomiting this morning. This is worse with moving her head from side to side. Her exam is normal except for some lateral nystagmus (twitching of the eyes when shifting from side to side) that is common with inner ear problems. Her work-up is unremarkable. The patient likely has a viral labrynthitis (inflammation of the inner ear), and responds to symptomatic medicines. The diagnosis I always at least consider in folks with these symptoms, is a stroke involving the posterior circulation of the brain. It can have similar symptoms, but is unlikely to respond to medicines for simple vertigo. I see one every few years. It usually presents much more dramatically, and they are typically progressively sicker.

At the same time as our 87-year-old, we have an uncomfortable 22-year-old Hispanic male complaining of three days of tooth pain. He speaks no English so requires a translator. He has a cavity you could drive a Mac truck into.

I don't understand why folks don't take care of dental problems before it becomes a crisis. I also don't understand why they choose the

Emergency Department to seek their dental care. Well, actually, I know why. Dentists usually want cash in advance in these cases, and have no obligation to see a patient otherwise. The Emergency Department must see everyone regardless of their means. Of course the ER bill is likely to be a lot more than the dentist might charge, but the ER bill is usually uncollectible.

I get this patient a course of antibiotics and some pain pills. I try to impress on him that he needs to see a dentist. It can be frustrating because the antibiotic often takes care of the underlying infection and the pain goes away. Then they don't see the dentist, and wind up back in here with the same complaint.

There seems to be growing numbers of Hispanics in the area. Most that we see speak little or no English (or want you to think that).

I realize that this last caveat might seem prejudicial, but I've lost track of the number of times my Hispanic patients suddenly understand English when it is convenient for them. I don't understand why, but it just happens a lot.

Many of the Hispanics use the Emergency Department to obtain all of their health care for themselves and their family. They like the convenience, because they don't want to have to be off work. They also know that we are required to see them.

The Hispanics also bring their own brand of social problems. Many of the young males seem to attempt to resolve their disputes with knives, and we see a fair number of stabbings. I wonder if this may be a changing trend, as we've recently seen more shootings. This is so much fun-Not.

So much for that diatribe. Next is a 50-year-old white female who was brought in by squad after she had a seizure. She has a history of a seizure disorder, and so this by itself isn't really cause for alarm. Her seizure has resolved spontaneously, and she was post-ictal (a post seizure state) by the time I see her. We check her seizure medicine levels to ensure they are adequate, and they are. We watch her for a while until she returns to baseline and then send her home. With a breakthrough seizure like this, she may need to be changed to a different medicine. She can follow-up with her neurologist to discuss this option.

Then I see a 32-year-old white female with alleged back pain after carrying an entertainment center. She tells me that her medical insurance doesn't start till tomorrow, and so her regular doctor-to-be told her to come here. Oh joy. It doesn't help that the only thing she isn't 'allergic' to is Vicodin (a oral narcotic). This sets off some alarm bells in my head. Ah well, my shift is almost over, and I'm feeling generous, so I gave her a few.

This is followed by a flurry of activity. I get a 74 year old white male who is unsteady on his feet, and an 89 year old while male with newly diagnosed atrial fibrillation who has been having increasing shortness of breath for the last week....But, my relief is here. After a quick checkout, I am out of here. These can all be someone else's problem. Yesss...

And so ends my 24 hour workday.

12:00 PM

Shift 2
"You've got me confused with someone who gives a damn!"

Saturday—18 Hours

Noon

Well a new shift has started. It's noon on a Saturday and this means the local doctors offices are just closing. The prior shift is finishing up two patients, so I won't have to see them. It's a clean slate, but there's one just checking in. Eighteen hours and counting.

I frequently tell my wife that going to work is a lot like going to war. I just do it on a schedule is all. You never know what is going to walk through your door, and on a weekend, the floodgates seem to be wide open. It can really be draining.

First call of the day is a 4-month-old Hispanic male whose parent thinks "feels hot". He's been fussy, and they also think he might have a red eye. Of course, this is essentially a well baby check. The child does not have a fever. His exam is normal, and his eye is fine. If anything, the child may have a virus, but even that is a stretch. Tylenol as needed is all that's needed at this time, if at all.

Next is a 57 year old white female with intermittent angioedema (facial soft tissue swelling) for the last 10 years. She'd had another outbreak this morning and has taken some Atarax (an antihistamine) when the symptoms started, but they persist. She is in no distress, and is having no shortness of breath (sometimes severe angioedema can obstruct the airway). She's had a complete work-up in the past with no specific findings. She presents for evaluation and treatment because the symptoms are not resolving as quickly as they have in the past.

Angioedema is typically allergy mediated. There tend to be high levels of histamine in the body, and it is this that produces the symptoms. As such, it is typically initially treated with antihistamines. When this doesn't work, steroids are often added. The final approach to treatment is H^2 blockers (Zantac, Pepcid, etc); these medicines also act at histamine receptors and can provide some additional symptomatic improvement.

Again, this lady has minimal symptoms, so I put her on a Prednisone taper (an oral steroid), and she can follow-up as needed. These types of symptoms can sometimes take days to resolve, so I give her a six day course of the medicine.

The patients are starting to stack up. This is the implication of my prior comment about the doctor's offices. When they close, it's like the flood gates open and people begin pouring into the Emergency Department.

I have an 11-year-old white male who cut his left arm on a piece of metal at the local fairgrounds. It's a minor injury that is easily repaired. Three sutures, tetanus shot, and he is out the door.

Then I have a 6-year-old white male who is listed as having "possibly" hurt his left great toe on a trampoline last night. Apparently his mother hadn't even looked at the toe in question. He has an abscess as big as my thumb that looks to have been festering for some time. Somehow I don't think it's related to the trampoline debacle. Ya think? I open it with a scalpel and get a nice rush of pus. It showed gram-positive cocci on the gram stain (a stain used to both make bacteria more visible under the microscope, and to help identify them), and was sent for culture. These wounds are usually infected with skin surface bacteria (typically gram positive) that have been tracked into the deeper tissues. An antibiotic active against the most probable organisms is all the more that's needed, and he's good to go. The best thing I've done for him is to drain the abscess. Antibiotics don't do a very good job of penetrating pus.

Then we have a surprisingly common problem, a 76-year-old white male with a terminal lung cancer. He'd been getting radiation therapy, but didn't tolerate the adjuvant chemotherapy; it suppressed his bone marrow so much that he became very anemic. The patient and his family have no insight into the fact that his condition is fatal. The patient looks miserably depressed.

Unless these tumors can be resected for cure, the prognosis is grim. There is around a 10-15% one year survival rate. Chemo and radiation are strictly palliative, but the radiation therapy is more effective if chemotherapy is also given.

This gentleman has had decreased oral intake and weakness. His family is concerned that he is just not getting better. And guess what? He's not going to get a lot better. I explain the lung cancer facts of life (and death) to the patient and his family in a manner they can best understand and deal with.

A big component is cases like this is reactive depression. We as a society deal poorly with issues of mortality. I impressed on this patient that he needs to try and do things he finds enjoyable, to eat anything that might taste good, and to make the very best of whatever time he has left. It is sad that patient's regular physicians so often do such a poor job of telling them they are going to die. Hope is one thing, but people sometimes need to know to make preparations for the end.

In the case of this patient, the family really resonated with what I had to say. They vocalize a renewed intent to be proactive about involving the patient and getting him to see other family members and the like. I think this is likely to be better for him than any prescription I could write.

Seems like we're running a cancer ward here. The next patient is a 53-year-old white female with recurrence of a breast cancer. She has been getting chemotherapy and was found to have a low white count in her doctor's office today. She was sent over for a shot of Neupogen (an immune system stimulant) to be given today and tomorrow. If her numbers can't be bolstered she faces increasing risk of fortuitous infection.

The Emergency Department has an outpatient role, especially on the weekends, and we give recurring shots and IVs as directed by patients regular doctors. In this patient, this is an expected complication of the chemotherapy. Many of these agents have very predictable time frames where a patient's white cell count reaches its low point, or nadir. She is right on time for the agent she's on. She's given her Neupogen and sent on her way.

Geriatrics to pediatric, next is an 8-year-old white male who had re-injured a great toe that had been lacerated a week previously. The family is spazzing out because it is bleeding slightly. The wound is still significantly intact, and has broken open just enough to get some trace bleeding. It just needs a Band-Aid.

Then I see a 12-year-old white male who had been struck on the forehead the night before with a block of 2X4 that had been winged at him by a sibling. There had been no loss of consciousness, and he had done fine since. He was brought in because there was a persistent swelling where the block of wood had struck him. Here again, you just scratch you head at the lack of both forethought and common sense. He has a small hematoma (collection of blood under the tissue) on his forehead. He'll have a bruise, and it'll get better on its own. He is out of here.

Then we're back to geriatrics and a 76-year-old white female with slurred speech, left facial droop, and difficulty walking for the last 6 hours. This is likely a TIA (transient ischemic accident) or stroke. There's been a lot of new coverage of the use of TPA (tissue plasminogen activator, a clot busting drug) in the use of stroke, but it's got to be given within the first 3 hours of onset of symptoms, so this patient doesn't qualify. A CT scan of her head is normal, so it is unlikely that her symptoms are due to a bleed. It's likely she has had a small blood clot lodge in her brain. Her deficit is not significant, and showed some improvement while we were evaluating her. Since she continued to have active symptoms, her regular doctor was contacted. He took over the case, and the patient was admitted.

Back into the fray with a 40-year-old white female who cut her right thumb on a piece of glass. It's pretty superficial. There's no tendon or nerve involvement. Two sutures and she is fixed.

Then an 11-year-old white female who fell out of the pear tree she was climbing. She has a left ear laceration and a left shoulder abrasion. A little Dermabond (skin glue) and she is right as rain.

I keep moving room to room.

Next is a 55-year-old white male who lacerated his right eyebrow on the sharp edge of a ladder jack. Six sutures and he is gone.

Then there is a 13-year-old white male who jumped off of the couch at home. He has right foot pain. The nurses know to just go ahead and get X-rays before I even see patients like this. He winds up with a 5th metatarsal fracture (a bone on the outside of the foot, and a common site of injury). After discussion with his regular doctor, he gets a walking boot, and the recommendation to follow-up first of the week.

Next is the worried well. It's an 85-year-old white female with increased blood pressure for the last couple of days. She had just been started on a new arthritis medicine, Vioxx. This is known to produce hypertension as a side effect in a small number of patients. I stop her Vioxx, switch her to a medicine less likely to produce this effect. She is going to see her regular doctor the first of the week, so she can have her blood pressure rechecked again at that time.

Pre-dinner rush, and I see a 6-year-old with sore throat, ear pain and fever. He got a positive rapid strep test, and so has strep throat. Antibiotics will help him.

Dinner is pathetic in the hospital cafeteria. The best I can manage is a hot dog.

6:00 PM

Next is a 6-year-old white female who cut her right hand with a knife at home. Her father brought her in. He said, "It's not very deep and it probably just needs a Band-Aid, but we wanted to have it looked at just the same. It's free." This is a typical attitude of our Medicaid patients that we see in the Emergency Department. Of course it's not free. You and I pay for it. This was hardly more than a scratch. Even a Band-Aid was overkill. She's out of here. Too bad I can't write a script for new parents.

This is followed by a 2-year-old white female who's had increased fussiness through the day. She has a bright red right ear drum but otherwise has no localizing findings. It looks like an otitis media (ear infection). Antibiotics should make it better.

Back to geriatrics and a 69-year-old white female with transient tingling of her left hand while getting down the dishes. She has a history of atrial fibrillation (an irregular heartbeat that can predispose one to stroke), and is on Coumadin (a blood thinner) to reduce stroke risk. Of course, she is concerned about stroke, but has no symptoms at presentation. Given the blood thinner, it is reasonable to scan her head to make sure she's not had a bleed. It's also reasonable to check and see how thin the Coumadin has made her blood. The work-up begins…

In the meantime we get a 30-year-old white male who slid into a base while playing baseball. He complains of right knee pain and swelling. There has been no other specific trauma. His exam reveals some minimal soft tissue swelling, and is otherwise normal. The patient is sure his leg was broken. This is very improbable given the mechanism of injury, but an X-ray is done just the same, and of course it is normal. This is a simple sprain that the average person would have treated at home. Rest, ice, elevation, an Ace wrap, and an anti-inflammatory like Motrin or Aleve are all that's needed.

Then we have a 39-year-old white obese female with intermittent nausea, vomiting and right upper quadrant pain for a month. These symptoms recurred tonight after a large meal. She has focal pain and tenderness under the ribs on the right. She was scheduled for an ultrasound later in the week to rule out gallbladder disease, but she feels she just can't wait any longer. We give her some Toradol (an anti-inflammatory medicine), some Compazine (a nausea medicine), and start our evaluation…

We get the scan and laboratory results back on our 69-year-old with the tingling left hand, and it's all just fine. This could just as easily be some early carpal tunnel changes (narrowing in the canal in the wrist that the median nerve goes through, that produces hand and arm numbness), or even a complete nothing. She is on the most aggressive treatment for stroke prevention that there is, and so we really have little to offer except for reassurance. She can follow-up with her regular doctor.

Then we're back to pediatrics and an 8-year-old white male who took a fall at the local swimming pool. He complains of right lower leg pain and is unable to bear weight. An X-ray demonstrates a right mid-shaft tibia fracture (the big bone in the lower leg). A call to the orthopedic surgeon takes the case out of my hands. Given the appearance of the fracture, this might require surgery to fix.

One of the highest litigated emergency room cases is orthopedic problems, and missed fractures. This is why almost everything that could possibly include a boney injury is X-rayed, regardless of the likelihood of a positive finding. Actually a large number of tests in the Emergency Department, perhaps as many as 80-90% are strictly medico-legal. Until there is massive reform of medical liability law, this is not likely to change. It only takes one lawsuit to really ruin your day (or career, or life for that matter)!

Back to the 39-year-old with the nausea, vomiting, and right upper quadrant pain. Everything is normal, including the ultrasound. She does not have gallstones like she thought. Also, her symptoms have completely resolved. This makes it more likely it is just a stomach bug, irritable bowel, or some other more benign process case. It warrants symptomatic treatment for now. She can follow-up with her regular doctor, and he can pursue it further as he sees fit.

Next is a 64-year-old white male with two weeks of left ankle pain. It is no better or worse today than any other day in the last two weeks, but now is the time he wants it checked out. The patient is a diabetic. His films are normal. He has focal tenderness on the inside of the ankle. This is a point of attachment of ligaments. There is no evidence of infection or inflammation. Despite no recalled trauma, this is most consistent with an ankle sprain. Routine care is warranted. He was given an Air Splint he can wear in his shoe, and put on some Daypro (an anti-inflammatory).

Then we have a 19-year-old white female requesting a pregnancy test. She has been sexually active and is not using any form of birth control. She wonders if she may be pregnant. Her last period was about a month ago. She is having no symptoms. She hasn't bothered to either get an over-the-counter test or see her regular doctor. When you're on welfare you can get free medical care whenever you want. No she's not pregnant, thankfully. She is counseled about safe sex and birth control, but she really isn't very interested in either.

9:00 PM

Time for the before bedtime rush…This time of night everyone seems to come in at once. Typically folks have had symptoms for some time, but as bedtime gets closer, they suddenly reach crisis stage.

It's interesting how there is a similar effect observed just after a big football game on TV. During the game it's okay, but after the game is over, its time to race to the ER.

Well, time for rapid-fire medicine. The nurses are lining them up so I can expedite the cases.

First an 8-year-old white female that was being chased by other children. She tripped over a teeter totter and struck her chest. She also bit her tongue. She has bumps bruises and a superficial tongue abrasion. Ice chips, Tylenol, and Motrin are the order of the day. We did a chest X-ray just because her mom felt she hit the ground "so hard," and insisted that we do so. Of course the films were normal. This is what we know as therapeutic X-rays.

The most unpleasant thing about doing pediatric medicine is dealing with the parents. Almost universally, at least in the ER setting, they have no insight into what constitutes something to worry about. They are so often sure that their child has some deadly disease if their child has had a fever for couple of hours, or a cough for a couple of days. Many of these children are constantly on antibiotics, really more to appease the parents rather than anything real. It is very frustrating, and the children suffer for it.

Second is a 9-year-old white male who cut his right index finger with a skinning knife. The tendon is intact. A few sutures and he was on his way.

Third is a 2-year-old white female with a few hours of a low grade fever (aha, what did I say). Her lab was normal, as is her exam. She is smiling, happy, and all better after Tylenol (what a magical drug. Too bad more parents don't know about it). If anything, she's got a little virus. I try and talk parents into symptomatic treatment where appropriate, and sometimes they'll go along with it. In this case they did, although they seemed skeptical.

Another reason some of the kids like this wind up inappropriately on antibiotics is the insecurity of the doctor. He might be worried about missing something, and if there were a problem that came to litigation, he could say, "well I had treated her aggressively and put her on an antibiotic…" I'll be the first to admit that American medicine routinely over-treats, especially in the ER setting.

Fourth is a 20-year-old white male from the local rodeo. He fell from a horse and lacerated his right upper eyelid. A few stitches and he is on his way, although this was not without a lot of fuss about having to use a needle. It just amazes me how big macho men are such wimps about shots and needles.

Fifth was a 58-year-old white female with 1 to 2 hours of left-hand pain and tenderness. She has no other focal symptoms. She has worked herself into a panic and hyperventilated. She is convinced that it is a heart attack. Of course, her work-up is normal, and her symptoms were cured with

Toradol (an anti-inflammatory medicine) and Ativan (a tranquilizer). She had had multiple work-ups in the recent past for similar symptoms. They were all normal. I have seen her many times in the past, and she is a nut with a capital "N". She leaves happy in the end after getting an hour or so of our attention. Who knows, maybe she has carpal tunnel, maybe she just had a spasm. At least she's out of my hair.

So frequently in the ER, especially in the evening, patients have huge psychiatric components. I've made tallies on many occasions, and typically get 80-90% of patients between midnight and 6 AM with significant psychiatric issues. Typically there is depression, anxiety and the like. Go figure…

Sixth is a 21-year-old white male who twisted his right knee two days ago. He had taken nothing for discomfort and had not attempted to be seen by his regular doctor even though offices were open yesterday and this morning. After the normal X-ray that he had requested, he was treated for his sprain with and air splint and an anti-inflammatory medicine.

Seventh is a 33-year-old white male that fell off a horse at the local rodeo. Do you see a pattern here? He sustained a right small finger fracture. It looks pretty nasty and is likely to need surgery to fix. Why is it that none of these folks who perform in these dangerous events like the rodeo ever have insurance. The orthopedic surgeon was called and assumed care. The cost to fix this guy's finger is likely to be a whole lot more than he makes in any ten rodeos.

Eighth, is a 37-year-old white male who had a tire explode in his face at the local demolition derby. He presented with eye pain and ringing ears. He has a big corneal abrasion on his right eye, and that eye is dilated and patched. The left was treated with antibiotic eye drops. He is given a pain medicine with instructions to follow-up.

These types of injuries usually heal on their own in 24 to 36 hours. Most of the pain and light sensitivity is from spasm of the muscle that controls the pupil. That's why we sometimes dilate the eye.

Ninth is a 36-year-old white male who was using a weed-whacker at home earlier in the day, and since that time has had increasing right eye pain. His exam reveals a large corneal abrasion. Okay, we need a third eye injury to satisfy our rule that these things come in threes. He is treated with antibiotic drops and pain medicine.

Tenth is 42-year-old white male with a scalp laceration. He was accidentally kicked in the head by a friend. Hmm, some friend. A few stitches and he is gone.

It's 10:00 PM and patients are still coming fast and furious. Hard to believe I've seen ten patients in the last hour. I'd like to see them do that in the average doctors office. Well time to get back to the madness…

Eleventh is a 38-year-old white female who was kicked in her right arm by a horse. Surprisingly this was not at the rodeo. She complains of upper arm pain. Her films are normal, and there is no evidence of a compartment syndrome (swelling in a compartment in the arm). In the end it's just a lot of bruising, and can be treated symptomatically.

Twelfth is a 55-year-old white female with five days of a posterior headache and some mattering of her right eye. She has a history of muscle tension headaches and that is what this seems to be. There is nothing to suggest a meningitis. I think it was the eye drainage that was the straw that broke the camel's back and brought her to the ER. Still, she does have a local doctor that she hasn't bothered to contact. Toradol (an anti-inflammatory) and Valium (a tranquilizer used as a muscle relaxant) cure her muscle tension headache. She is put on some antibiotic eye drops and goes home happy.

12:00 AM

Thirteenth is a 19-year-old white female who injured her right foot on a trampoline much earlier in the day. I see more injuries on these damn things. She has a small hematoma (collection of blood under the skin) on the top of her foot. The real agenda is that she doesn't want to have to work in the morning. I give her the get-out-of-jail-free card that she wants.

Just in general, so many people come into the emergency room with a specific agenda. Part of whether they leave happy, and don't write nasty letters to the hospital president, is figuring out what that agenda is. Then, of course, you need to decide if you can give them what they want without violating medical standards of care and the like. Many times they have completely unreasonable requests, and you just have to accept that it's going to generate a complaint. Life's a bitch.

Oh joy, fourteenth is a 30-year-old white male with four episodes of diarrhea over an hour. He's sure this has made him dehydrated. The agenda, again, is a get out of work card. Whatever...

Fifteenth is a 38-year-old white male with 4 days of fever, productive cough, pain with a deep breath, and shortness of breath. He does have a fever. His oxygen level is normal. Chest X-ray shows pneumonia in the upper part of his left lung. We got some cultures just in case he doesn't get better with the antibiotic I select. I then put him on Levaquin (a broad-spectrum antibiotic) plus something for pain. Tincture of time and he should do fine. Again, he's got a doctor...I'm starting to sound like a broken record.

Sixteenth is a 16-year-old crazy white female. She allegedly slipped in some grease at her place of employment and bumped her knee and head. This gave her one of her migraine headaches. She took her migraine medicine and developed abdominal pain. I'm always very suspicious of folks who are on 6 to 8 psychiatric medicines, and she fits the bill. Her evaluation was normal and she was cured with a GI Cocktail (Maalox and Viscous Lidocaine) and Zantac (a stomach acid reducer). Maybe her migraine medicine irritated her stomach. She actually left happy, thank God.

2:00 AM

If things are going to slow down a bit, this is normally the time it does. Usually on the weekends though it just keeps going through the night. I nip off to grab 2 or 3 winks, and...

Zzzz…

Amazing, three hours without a patient. I get to sleep.

As I had said before, one thing about medicine is that you have to learn to sleep when and how you can. There's no telling when you are going to have the opportunity. I've gotten so I can sleep pretty much anywhere, any time.

5:00 AM wake-up call is a 48-year-old white male who was kicked by a horse three days ago. He's been having right-sided rib pain that's just not getting better. Why 5:00 AM? Who knows. He's having no shortness of breath, or any other significant symptoms. His chest X-ray does show several broken ribs. This is treated symptomatically. Some pain pills he's gone. Of course he will have pain for the next two months till the ribs heal. The real risk here is a secondary pneumonia if his rib pain is not well enough controlled that he doesn't take good deep breaths.

6:00 AM

The boss is here taking a shift, nothing to pass off, so I am out of here…

Shift 3
"Stomping out disease and pestilence!"

Monday—18 Hours

6:00 PM

Well I've been off a whopping 36 hours. Somehow it feels like I've never even left. There was one patient left from the last shift, but the previous doc stayed around long enough to finish it up. So starts my 18-hour sojourn.

Of course the doctors offices are closed now, so the local populace will stew for awhile, and then start coming in en-masse. Mondays are frequently every bit as bad as the weekends. Those folks who tried to hold out to see their regular doctor after the weekend, often find that they are not able to get in until later in the week. They tend to lose their patience.

Well, I've hardly been on duty five minutes and we have an 82-year-old white female with a rash after working in the garden. It's been present 4-5 days and an emergency tonight. She has a local doctor, but didn't bother to try and contact him. She has a contact dermatitis, probably poison ivy, on her arms and around her eye. The eye itself is not involved. She wants a shot to cure it. I give her a shot of Decadron (a steroidal anti-inflammatory) and

Vistaril (an antihistamine). This will help, but probably won't cure it by itself, so I put her on some oral meds as well.

Well true to form, I've been here half an hour, and the waiting room is starting to fill up. On the scanner it sounds like a squad is heading out to pick up our city's ill and down-trodden. The call was for a medical emergency, but more times as not it's just a sick call in need of a taxi ride.

But first I have a 12-year-old white female who twisted her right ankle. The X-ray is normal. She just has a sprain. She gets my standard treatment of ice, air splint, elevation, anti-inflammatories, weight bearing as tolerated, and follow-up as needed. I need a stamp for these, they are so routine.

Second I see a 20-month-old white female with two days of a progressive rash. It's much worse today. It looks like chicken pox (caused by the Veracella zoster virus) with little vesicles (water blisters). The child did have a chicken pox vaccination, but who knows how well her immune system responded to it. Symptomatic treatment is in order.

And the squad arrives. It's a 47-year-old white male with chest pain. Oh joy, there are lots of psychiatric overtones. The patient had been trying to get disability for diffuse pain complaints. As expected, the ER work-up was negative. He did have a normal stress test two years ago. He still needs a cardiac evaluation, especially given the disability angle. This would be one who would sue in a heartbeat if you missed something. The on-call doctor doesn't want to keep him for this. He says he'll be in much later to reevaluate the patient. We'll see…

Fourth, and Oh boy, my favorite (Not), a 59-year-old white female with a migraine headache since the afternoon. She hasn't taken anything for it since it started, but that doesn't stop her from coming to the emergency room as we get close to bedtime. I give her one of the headache concoctions (Nubain, Phenergan, DHE45) she has had before and she goes away.

Fifth we have a 5-year-old white male who was allegedly sexually fondled by another boy of about the same age. The police are involved. There was no probability of sexual penetration. This becomes more of a civil matter.

Sixth is a 43-year-old white female with fever, body aches, cough, and back pain through the day. She does have quite an elevated white blood count. Otherwise everything is normal. I'll cover her with an antibiotic just because the lab numbers make me nervous. I get blood cultures first. She can follow-up with her regular doctor.

Seventh is a 5-year-old white male with poison ivy. He had it just a week ago, but now it's back. Steroids and antihistamines are the medicines of the day it seems.

Eighth we have a 60-year-old white male with chest pressure for an hour. He had two of his wife's nitroglycerine with complete resolution of his symptoms. He is an adult onset diabetic and has refractory hypertension. He's also a smoker. If he doesn't have coronary artery disease, he sure deserves it. He's got some nonspecific EKG changes, otherwise his ER work-up is unremarkable. We get him admitted early so he can be ruled out and get a stress test.

Ninth, Fast and furious, is a 18-year-old white male who hit the floor with his face while playing basketball. There was no loss of consciousness. He wound up with a left eyebrow laceration out of it, gets some stitches, and is out of here.

Tenth we have a 20-year-old white female with a two day history of fever, nausea, vomiting, and diarrhea. Her mom has similar symptoms that started at the same time. Her mother had gotten dehydrated to the point where she had needed some IV fluids. The daughter figures she needs some too. Like mother, like daughter, ya think? Of course there is no objective evidence that the daughter is at all dehydrated. This is McMedicine though, service with a smile, so we give her a liter of fluid and she goes away happy.

Eleventh is a 17-month-old white female who had vomited three times after waking up. Her mother felt she "looked pale" and "seemed confused". Of course the child is smiling, happy, playful, and in no distress whatever. Her exam is completely normal. I try to provide some reassurance, but who knows how well I get through. This is pediatrics, remember?

Twelfth is a 2-month-old white female with five episodes of vomiting over a couple of hours. Do you see a trend here? It's the same chapter and verse. This just requires supportive care. This mom needed therapeutic lab studies just to prove everything was okay. She seems reassured in the end.

Thirteenth is a little odd. It is a 32-year-old white female who was brought in by her family with "confusion". She was no sooner in the room when the family demands, "well, you're going to admit her aren't you?" I have to explain, once again, that one of the roles of the Emergency Room is to assess whether that is necessary, but that it is pretty hard to determine that in 15 seconds.

This woman had been in the night before with complaints of weakness and shortness of breath. She had had laboratory that suggested dehydration to the physician on duty at the time. Otherwise, he wasn't able to find much else wrong. It had been recommended that she get more fluids.

The (unspoken, unwritten) rules of the game are, if a patient returns, you should do more than the previous visit. So I pull out the stops and ordered a full battery of tests. In the meantime I start re-hydrating the patient. We'll see what we find...

Fourteenth, I have a 61-year-old white female with a three-week history of neck pain. Several years ago she had been told she had a thyroid problem, but she had not followed up with that as she didn't have insurance. Her lab is normal, but she has a mass on chest X-ray. This looks like a lung cancer. She is a big smoker so she does have a pretty good risk factor. You draw your own conclusions. Unless it's resectable, the one-year survival rate is 10-15%. This doesn't require admission. She can follow-up outpatient for the evaluation.

Fifteenth, we have a 16-month-old white female that touched a hot lamp and burned the tips of two fingers. You can barely see two little red spots if you use your imagination. Why this required me to look at it I don't know. The most it might need is a Band-Aid, if that.

Sixteenth, oh joy, a 22-year-old white female who's 2 months pregnant. She had some cramping after sex, and is sure something is wrong with the baby. She also started having diarrhea today. Of course, everything is normal, but she really wants an ultrasound. I'm able to justify it to rule out an ectopic pregnancy (a fetus where it doesn't belong, like in the fallopian tubes), but only just barely. Of course, the ultrasound is normal, and the fetus looks fine. It looks like she just has a little stomach bug. Again, symptomatic medicines are the rule of the day.

Seventeenth, (again, the later is gets, the more psychiatric overtones I deal with) is a 29-year-old white female having a panic attack. She took two of her Xanax (a tranquilizer), but still couldn't calm down. Well take two more! I gave her an injected equivalent that mellowed her out. She has more psychiatric issues than you can shake a stick at, but I'm not going to solve them in my Emergency Room. I recommend that she consider getting some counseling. She's not very receptive to the idea. Oh well. You can lead a horse to water, etc, etc.

Follow-up on the 32-year-old confused woman. She is in progressive renal failure. She has a wide anion gap metabolic acidosis. This means that there is something in her blood making it more acidic. You can sometimes get this with renal failure and with diabetes, but the picture doesn't fit. The family confides that she is a BIG alcoholic. She must have ingested something. Antifreeze would do this. The patient denies it, but it's very suspicious. Well, we have more than enough to admit her. Maybe I'll find out what the real story is when I go to sign my dictated chart (I usually get these after the patient is discharged, transferred, or has died). She is admitted, and becomes someone else's problem.

Eighteenth, and we're back to the geriatric crowd. We have an 85-year-old white female who had heard a pop while bending a few days ago and has been experiencing left sided rib pain. She has no doctor. You can hardly even see her ribs on X-ray; her bones are so thin. I can't find it, but I'm pretty sure she has spontaneously fractured a rib or two. This is a lesson to women everywhere, drink your milk, go on replacement estrogen after menopause, and you will avoid such stuff. In this case all I have to offer is symptomatic treatment. She needs to get a regular doctor and consider evaluation for medicines to rebuild bone mass.

12:00 AM

Now its midnight, the witching hour has arrived. For the moment I see no sign of reprieve. Ah well, may as well get back to it.

Nineteenth, I see a 39-year-old white female with a one day history of a sore throat. She wants an antibiotic, so I give her one. I could do a strep screen to see if it is viral or bacterial. In adults it's usually viral, and not helped by antibiotics. What I'm faced with is that patients usually want an antibiotic anyway. So, in this case, I forgo the $100 test and give them what they want.

Well, surprise, surprise, I have a reprieve. Off I go to try and get some sleep.

Zzzz...

I do well to until about 1:30 AM. Then the phone rings with the announcement that multiple traumas are inbound. Shit, shit, shit...I hate trauma. We're just not set up for it. It takes a very proactive surgery staff, and the surgeons here just aren't very interested.

It seems a drunken kid drove a car through a group of people. Five traumas are inbound.

The first to arrive, I'm told is the worst. It's a 17-year-old white female with multiple injuries to include head injuries. She had been knocked unconscious at the scene, and had not fully recovered. She doesn't speak, but will obey commands. There are multiple lacerations, abrasions, and contusions. There are also obvious broken bones in the extremities. We get a chest and cervical spine X-ray, which look okay, and whisked her down to the X-ray department to get a head CT and more films. Meanwhile, more folks keep pouring in...

A 39-year-old white male was struck in the right shoulder in the event. His films are normal. He is just bruised. We treat him and street him.

A 16-year-old white female was struck in the left forehead in the event and has a left eyebrow laceration. There was no reported loss of consciousness, but she is having some problem with short term memory, so likely has a concussion. She also has multiple bumps and bruises. We scan her head and film everything that hurts, and are unable to find any significant injury. Her eyebrow is repaired, and she is released to the custody of her mother.

Back to the 17-year-old with head trauma. She becomes unresponsive in the radiology suite, and is obviously becoming more unstable. She's also more tachycardic and her blood pressure is dropping. Since this facility has no neurosurgical support, it's time to punt to the big boys. I contact the on-call trauma center and arrange to ship her pronto. The helicopter isn't flying due to thunder storms in the area, so we get ground transport mobilized. She is loaded and out the door.

In the middle of all of this we get a 39-year-old white female who injured her right little finger at work. It was a crush injury. She's managed a partial amputation of the finger. I call in the on-call orthopedic surgeon to deal with it. Then it's no longer my problem.

Back to the participants in the conflagration. There is a 17-year-old white male with multiple superficial cuts and scrapes and a large scalp laceration. We get him filmed, and then sew up his scalp. He goes home with his parents.

Then we have an 18-year-old Hispanic male whose left thigh was struck by a glancing blow. His evaluation doesn't reveal anything more than bruising, but he is having a hard time bearing weight on the leg. The orthopedic surgeon is still in the emergency room, and so I have him look at the patient. He concurs that there is no significant injury. In the end this patient gets observed over night just for good measure.

Wouldn't you know, as all of this craziness has been going on, there was a patient in the lobby demanding to be seen right away. She hadn't pooped in several days and was very uncomfortable. You know, with aisles and aisles of medicines in every drug store and grocery store to make you poop, I have yet to figure out why it warrants an emergency room visit without at least trying something. Ah well, mine is not to question why...

My evaluation didn't reveal anything else of note. She gets an enema, and goes home a lot lighter, with a smile on her face.

6:00 AM

True to form, folks with similar symptoms show up together. Next is a 66 year old white male with one week of low abdominal pain, worse this morning. This gentleman has a history of prostate cancer. He had had a radical prostatectomy (the surgical removal of his prostate gland due to prostate cancer) several years ago, but had had a recurrence, with at least one metastatic lesion present. This patient was in obvious discomfort. The true tale was told when I did a CT of his belly. He had pretty widely metastatic disease. He and his wife had little insight into just how dire his prognosis really was. I get him admitted, but his future looks grim.

Then we have a 19-year-old black male who had been vomiting through the morning, and noticed blood in what he had vomited. Of course the exam and the lab were normal. Just as we were about to place a NG (nasogastric tube to pump the stomach), he had a large emesis that was negative for blood. It isn't unusual with forceful vomiting, to irritate the esophagus and get some bleeding. It is usually minimal and self-limited. It all falls under the category of Mallory Weiss tear of the esophageal mucosa. I did go ahead and give this guy some IV fluids and anti-nausea medicines. Then I sent him on his way feeling better than when he had arrived.

9:00 AM

Back to my room then for a well needed nap. I am out until noon. Zzzz...

12:00 PM

Shift change and I am out of here. I finish my dictations and hit the road. As expected, as I was leaving, the lobby is filling up with yet more worried well patients clamoring to be seen. Not my problem...

Shift 4
"Don't go away mad.
Just go away!"

Wednesday—18 Hours

12:00 AM

Well hell, it seems like I only just left this place. Didn't I say that just last shift? You never know quite what to expect when you enter at the witching hour. The leaving physician tells me it should be slow (Uh oh the infamous "S" word not used by Emergency Room staffers) because he had just seen everyone in town. I know that sometimes it seems like that to me as well.

Well, let's see. What sort of worried well do we have to evaluate...?

My first case of the night is a 7-month-old white male with some redness of the end of his penis, actually more the foreskin. Allegedly the family have only noticed this evening. They are going on a road trip in the morning, and felt it should be checked before they go. Why they decided this at midnight, I can't fathom. Sometimes in these little guys they get some persistent adhesions from their circumcisions that trap some smegma and become inflamed. I don't see that in this case. I cover him with an antibiotic in case this is a little local infection, and will have them follow-up when they get back in a couple of days.

Then we have an 18-year-old white male with right foot pain. He had been wrestling yesterday and his friend said he heard a pop when he twisted his foot. He comes in with a bevy of little teenybopper girl friends that are fawning over him. Of course he's playing it up to the max. In the end, there's nothing really wrong with him, except perhaps a mild sprain. It could have been taken care of with some Motrin or Aleve. He hasn't tried either. Once again, why this is an emergency after midnight I don't know

Ah well, a short reprieve, and I'm off and napping.

Zzzz...

It's 2:00 AM and I see a little 2-year-old white female with left-sided abdominal pain. She's had recurrent problems with constipation, and had had a small hard stool two days prior. She had some focal left lower abdominal tenderness. A belly X-ray shows mega-poop. A pediatric fleets enema, and after much grunting, she gives birth to a huge turd. Symptoms resolved, and case cured. I also give her some MOM (Milk of Magnesia, a laxative) to ensure the job is completed. I recommended MOM as needed, increased fiber and the like.

Back to bed.

Zzzz...

It's just before 4:00 AM, and we get a 64-year-old white female with shortness of breath. She has known COPD (chronic obstructive lung disease) and was in a couple of days before with similar symptoms. She was started on some antibiotics, steroids, and breathing meds, but has been completely non-compliant with this. She also continues to smoke a pack or more a day despite her shortness of breath.

I just don't understand people who have such severe lung disease and don't make the association that it is either directly caused by, or at least exacerbated by, their cigarette smoking. They can be gasping for breath, but still sucking down one last cigarette. I routinely see folks with tobacco associated oral cancers who've wound up with permanent tracheostomies, breathing through their trachs. I also routinely see folks who have smoked themselves into such severe lung disease that they are on chronic supplemental oxygen and gasping for breath with any exertion; they continue to smoke while on oxygen. The power of denial is, if nothing else, very impressive.

Well, I have Respiratory give this woman several breathing treatment, and the nurse gives her a shot of some Decadron (a steroid). This brings her back to baseline. We encourage her to take the medicines as directed, and to at least cut back her smoking until her breathing is better. Who knows…?

My pillow is calling my name.

Zzzz…

6:00 AM

Time for my 6 o'clock wake-up call. An 88-year-old white female comes in by squad complaining of feeling weak for the last several days. She was just in to see her doctor yesterday. Today she just feels too weak. Of course every test we manage is completely normal. She strikes me as depressed. She lives alone, which may be a part of it. I chat with her doctor, and we have social services place her in a nursing home.

At the same time we get a 38-year-old white male with palpitations for an hour. He's had similar episodes in the past, but it's never lasted this long. He had been seen for it before, but never followed up. He's diaphoretic (sweaty), but otherwise is tolerating a 220 heartbeat very well. We give him two doses of Adenosine (a fast acting medicine that slows the heart) that converts him back to a sinus rhythm. I then give him some Lopressor (a longer acting rate control medicine) to keep him in a normal rhythm. This is not a threatening arrhythmia, so after a couple hours of observation, he is able to go with follow-up. Hopefully, this time he does follow up.

Next is a 78-year-old white female with known hemorrhoids, who had some blood in her stool after a bowel movement. This is something of a no brainer. I guess she did try and talk to her regular doctor about it, but he is off today. She has had a recent colonoscopy (a fiber-optic that evaluates the entire colon) that was unremarkable. On exam, she has some dried blood on a hemorrhoid, otherwise nothing. Her lab is otherwise normal. She went home with some hemorrhoid suppositories, and the recommendation to follow-up with her regular doctor.

Well, the scanner has the squad out on a male with a shoulder injury. We'll see what it is.

And it's a 46-year-old white male with spontaneous right shoulder pain and deformity. He has a history of spontaneous dislocation of his left shoulder in the past. There was no trauma with this event. His symptoms resolve when the patient is transferred from squad cart to ER cart prior to going to X-ray. He states that it felt like it 'popped back in'. We'll film it regardless.

At the same time we receive a 41-year-old white female who became lightheaded at work. She has been under a lot of stress for a couple of months, and has had multiple similar episodes. This was the worst in a while. Her evaluation is normal. This looks like a stress mediated vasovagal process. It's similar to what happens when you faint. Her anxiety is helped with Xanax (a tranquilizer). I recommend that she get some counseling to help with the stress. I also give her the day off, which is what she really seems to want.

Films are back on our shoulder guy. They are consistent with someone whose shoulder had been dislocated. He's put in a shoulder immobilizer with the recommendation that he see one of the orthopedic surgeons.

Lunchtime, and that means cafeteria mystery meat, reconstituted potato mash, and near liquid boiled carrots. Yum yum.

12:00 PM

Then we have a 59-year-old white male who was one of our old frequent fliers. He was quite the drug seeker, until he stopped getting what he wanted. He's had a cough for the last couple of days. He says he recently had pneumonia, and is worried about it coming back. His chest X-ray is unremarkable. He wants an antibiotic, so we put him on some Doxycycline for good measure. Why do I get the feeling that we are going to start seeing him again more frequently?

Next is an 11-year-old white male with pain and tenderness over his right eye. He has had quite a bit of sinus drainage. The pain was helped with Advil. Sounds most like a frontal sinusitis, although he may also have some allergies. I covered him with an antihistamine and an antibiotic. He can keep using the Advil, but based on his age and weight, he can take more than he has been getting.

It's time for the afternoon rush.

First is an 11-year-old white male with a right shin laceration. He crashed into a bike ramp with his bike. Of course he wasn't wearing a helmet or any other protective gear. He has no other injuries except the laceration. He is pretty skittish, but I get him calmed down enough to get him sewn up.

We hear the squad out on the scanner. A car drove into a trailer. Hmmm. Trauma? MI?

Turns out it is a 64-year-old white male who was stung by a bee while driving his car. He had an anaphylactic reaction, got hypotensive enough to lose vision transiently and drive off the road striking a trailer. He became slightly short of breath, and developed an itchy rash. There was no real damage to his car or the trailer. The squad was called, and they gave him some IV Benadryl (an antihistamine), and some IV fluids. He was pretty much symptom free at arrival, but I gave him some Decadron (a steroid) and some Zantac (a reflux medicine) for good measure.

Anaphylactic reactions like this are a type of allergic reaction, just like angioedema. These are mediated by histamine and are treated just the same.

This gentleman did well with it all. I recommended he talk with his regular doctor about an epinephrine pen. This is a portable kit you carry with you in case you get a bee sting somewhere that you are unable to get immediate attention.

Down time. Time for a nap.

Zzzz…

Well, that was a nice couple hour nap. It's 5:00 PM and the doctors' offices are closed. They should start to come in now…

And here we go. The first patient is a 68-year-old white male who just got out of the hospital. He has lung cancer that is metastatic to his brain. He has been getting radiation therapy and chemotherapy. His white count has been low and he was to get a Neupogen shot (an immune system stimulator). He stopped by the doctors' office, but they were not able to get the medicine so late in the day, so he was sent over here for this. The patient has no other issues. He was just seen in the office, and is going to be seen again in the morning for a recheck of his white count. We got him stabbed and out the door. Seems like a nice guy. Bad things even happen to nice guys.

Wow, I've had a serious brain fart. Somehow I was thinking my shift went to 8:00 PM. No, only until 6:00 PM. I'm almost out of here. Rather a pud shift in the scheme of things. I'm not due back till Saturday. Cool.

6:00 PM

Shift 5
"Lack of forethought on your part does not constitute a crisis on my part!"

Saturday—18 Hours

6:00 AM

Well we're off to a bad start. Everyone seems to be in a rather pissy mood today. The local doctors are dumping on one another, and don't want to take responsibility for the patients that they should. All in all, the start of what could be a really shitty day. Nursing shift change is in an hour. I hope that brings some improvement with it.

Holdovers include a 29-year-old white female with recurrent problems with hemarthrosis (bleeding into her knee). She's on a blood thinner for blood clots. The local orthopedic surgeon will be in eventually to look after her.

There were two others, but the doctor from the previous shift finished them before leaving.

Okay, now for the start of my day. First we have a 77-year-old white female in by squad with an 'allergic reaction'. She is visiting from out-of-state and has a history of chronic back pain. This was exacerbated by her recent trip. She was seen last evening and given a Nubain (mild non-narcotic pain medicine) shot and some Darvocet (another mild pain medicine formulation composed of Tylenol and propoxefen). After taking the Darvocet at home, she began having dizziness, nausea, and vomiting. She is convinced that this is an allergic reaction. In reality, these are the most common known side effects of this medicine. She's also complaining bitterly of her back pain.

True to the rule of "do more if they return", I'm filming her back, doing a range of lab, and getting her some fluids and meds to calm her stomach and back pain. This lady is dramatic to beat the band. It makes me wonder how much of this is supratentorial (psychiatric). We'll see…

Well it's not looking good. Another squad is inbound. An elderly 81-year-old white female coming in with back pain.

In the meantime, I have a 30-year-old white female who had been working at a new job for the last week where she is constantly on her feet. She complains of pain in the arches of her feet, foot swelling, and an ankle rash. The foot pain and ankle swelling are easily accounted for by her recent increased activity. The rash is on both ankles just above the sock line. This has got to be some type of contact dermatitis. She was likely exposed to some new chemical agent on her new job. There is nothing else noteworthy. She needs better shoes, and an anti-inflammatory like Aleve for her feet, and some topical steroid for her rash. This is clinic work. A reasonable person would have taken some Aleve, and tried the OTC hydrocortisone for the rash rather than racing to the ER. Why do I even bother to complain?

The squad arrived with an 81-year-old white female with right-sided back pain for the last day. She has a twenty-year history of recurrent back and hip pain for which she gets intermittent epidurals. She has a label of sacroileitus, an inflammation of the joint between sacrum and iliac bones in the pelvis. She says she hasn't done anything different. Of course she hasn't taken anything for this, but called the squad right away. She has local tenderness around the sacrum. We'll film the area and give her something for discomfort. I'm underwhelmed. I wonder when we'll see the next back pain. We need at least three...

Well speak of the devil. Another squad is inbound with a 48-year-old white male with right lower back pain.

Meanwhile, our 77-year-old back pain had blood in her urine and a calcified aorta, so we need to rule out a kidney stone and an aortic aneurysm. She'll get an ultrasound to rule out these things.

Our 81-year-old back pain complains of it being worse after being in X-ray. The films are fine. We give her something more for pain, and send her on her way.

Well the squad is here. It's a 48-year-old white male with known degenerative disc disease and chronic back pain. He was in route to his regular doctor with his back pain complaint. The drive made it worse, so he stopped and called the squad. This is rich.

Our 77-year-old back pain had a normal ultrasound. We treat her symptomatically, and she's out the door.

Meanwhile we have an 81-year-old white female with cold symptoms for 3-4 days. She has a history of asthma and pneumonia. She's worried about pneumonia. Her oxygen level is normal, as is her chest X-ray. Her symptoms were better with a breathing treatment despite not having a lot of wheezes. We'll cover her with an antibiotic for good measure, and put her on some breathing medicines.

Next is an 84-year-old white male with known coronary artery disease who had one hour of left sided chest pain that started while he was working around the house. He states that this is identical to the pain he had before he has his angioplasty. He's having no other symptoms, and has had no chest pain since his angioplasty, until now. His EKG shows evidence of a prior heart attack, but doesn't show anything active. His symptoms resolve within minutes of getting some supplemental oxygen. This is unstable angina until proven otherwise. We'll get routine cardiac lab, but this one's a keeper.

Meanwhile we have an 81-year-old white male with several days of left-hand swelling. He has no history of trauma. Exam shows soft tissue swelling, otherwise normal. We'll put him on an anti-inflammatory for a few days with follow-up

Our 84-year-old with chest pain has elevated cardiac enzymes. He remains pain free. He probably has a small infarction of the endocardium (inner lining of the heart). The lack of EKG changes places this in the category of non-Q wave myocardial infarction. He's put on a range of protective medicines and admitted for further evaluation.

Now is as good a time as any to say a few words about management of cardiac chest pain. I have talked earlier about stable angina, unstable angina, and acute myocardial infarction. Well what do you do about it all?

When a person comes in with chest pain there is an initial EKG and a review of their history and risk factors. It isn't always completely clear whether chest pain is cardiac or not. The goal is to try and decipher this and to minimize risk of a bad outcome regardless.

If there is a strong suspicion that a patient is having angina or unstable angina, there are a range of protective things that are done that have been shown to decrease risk of progression to infarction and associated injury of heart muscle tissue. A patient is usually given an aspirin; this acts as a blood thinner and reduces risk of spontaneous small blood clots that can precipitate a heart attack in a person with narrowed heart vessels. They are put on oxygen to maximize oxygen delivery to the heart. They are given nitroglycerine, which dilates blood vessels to improve coronary artery flow and reduce spasm. They are given beta-blockers that decrease the load on the heart by slowing it, reducing the effect of stress hormones by blocking their receptors. Finally, they are given a heparin-like compound which further acts to thin their blood and reduce risk of clot formation. Some or all of these interventions frequently produce a complete resolution of pain.

If a person is actually having a heart attack, the preceding is done, but in addition, they are evaluated for TPA (tissue plasminogen activator, or the clot busting drug). They may also need some morphine to help with pain and anxiety. These actions are usually enough to deal with the immediate risks in an acute heart attack. Rarely, they are not adequate, and in that case, the patient gets referred for emergent angioplasty. My facility does not have this ability, and so these patients are shipped to a larger hospital that offers these services. Sometimes, in these larger hospitals, angioplasty occurs in lieu of TPA, just because you can kill three birds with one stone: evaluate the coronary arteries, open blockages, and dilate stenotic arteries.

Back to the present, and time for the important things in life, lunch time. Institutional spaghetti, oh joy.

12:00 PM

Then back into battle. We have a 40-year-old white male with increasing umbilical pain for the last 4 days. He seems to have a small hernia there that he states is new. It's all very unusual. This is something you normally see in children. He's had no abdominal surgeries that would predispose to a surgical hernia. I start a routine abdominal pain work-up and call the surgeon to come take a look.

Meanwhile I see a 19-year-old white male who was in a motor vehicle accident last night. He's now complaining of right foot pain. There was little pain initially. This hurts with walking and weight bearing. His exam and X-rays are normal. It's a bruise or sprain. Ice, elevate, compression, anti-inflammatories, pain control, and out the door.

With our umbilical pain gentleman, it has taken forever to get hold of the surgeon, but we finally did. We'll see. I had been getting ready to do a CT scan through his belly. The big concern would be an incarceration. This is rather unusual in a patient this age with no prior surgical history, but could happen…

The surgeon finally shows up and thinks that it is an incarcerated umbilical hernia. He'll take him to surgery later in the afternoon.

Next is a 78-year-old white female with a recent surgery for colon cancer. She was started on chemotherapy in the last week. Since then she has had nausea, diarrhea and abdominal cramping, and she wants something to stop the cramps. This has been going for a week, and the symptoms are unchanged. She just can't take it any longer. We start some fluids and gave her some Zofran (an IV anti-nausea medicine that works best with chemotherapy-associated nausea and vomiting). We also start an abdominal pain work-up to ensure nothing else is going on.

Then we have a 22-year-old white male who had fallen asleep at the wheel last night and wrecked his car. He complains of shoulder pain. The films are fine. He just has some bruising and superficial abrasions. This is treated symptomatically.

We also have a 19-year-old white male diabetic who had a low blood sugar at work. With this he had transient decreased vision, and was worried he would pass out. He took some candy, but then got panicky. He hyperventilated and scared his employer. They called the squad, and he was brought over. He was fine by the time he arrived. This is a common problem that rarely needs an ER visit. We fed him, watched him a while, rechecked his blood sugar, and sent him on his way.

Meanwhile, the next squad is just rolling in. It's a 79 year old white female with recurrent epigastric pain and burning. She's also had burning in the back of her throat for several days. This is better with belching and Maalox. She also has intermittent shortness of breath that she says occurs just when she gets up suddenly; she's had this for years. She states that she has a "heart history," but is unable to elaborate. She is planning on attending a wedding at the end of the week, and so feels she should get this looked at so it doesn't interfere with her plans. I get an EKG, normal. Old records are called for, and she's given some Maalox.

Meanwhile, there's a 59-year-old white male who had tripped over some uneven concrete and fallen on his outstretched left arm. He's complaining of pain in that wrist. An X-ray reveals a distal radius fracture. He's mashed the end of the long bone at the base of the thumb. He's managed to split it as well, and there's a crack extending into the joint. I call the orthopedic boys, and they take over for me.

Back to our 79-year-old with the chest burning. Her records show a history of intermittent atrial fibrillation. Her shortness of breath with rising has been present and unchanged for years. She's had several unremarkable cardiac work-ups. She is cured with Maalox, and the discomfort stays away with Zantac (a stomach acid lowering medicine). I think this is one that can be handled with outpatient follow-up.

It's always a difficult call. Of course the one you don't want to miss is an atypical presentation of cardiac chest pain. With as much as chest pain has been publicized in the media, we are frequently swamped with every little chest ache and twinge. If they were all admitted, the hospital would be overflowing. You really have to play out a combination of the risk factors, objective findings, intuition, plus a measure of medico-legal. It's when you get the weird ones, like a twenty-nine year old who really is having an infarct, that you get real nervous. Also, as I've said earlier, I've lost track of the number of times my intuition that something wasn't quite right has saved my butt.

Next is a 39-year-old white male who slid his arm against the sharp edge of a newly cut piece of pipe. He sustained a rather innocuous little forearm laceration, perhaps two inches long, but it is just spraying a continuous quarter inch stream of blood. This is one where you put a finger in the dike and let a surgeon take care of it. He is taken to the surgery suite for the repair.

Then we're back to the cancer wards with a 78-year-old white female who had advanced colon cancer. She had the tumor resected, and had been on chemotherapy for about a week. This whole time she has been having continuous problems with nausea, anorexia, diarrhea, and diffuse abdominal cramping. Our evaluation showed some decreased potassium, as was expected with diarrhea, and some mild dehydration. Otherwise, this appears to be just routine side effects of the chemo. We give her some fluids, anti-nausea medicine, and a mild pain medicine. In addition, we supplement her potassium. This gets her feeling a whole lot better in short order. She is able to go home with some symptomatic medicines and potassium supplementation. She already has follow-up scheduled for Monday.

Oh joy, more dentistry. A 24-year-old white female with one day of right jaw pain. No history of trauma. No other symptoms. She does grind her teeth at night and still has her wisdom teeth. There is no tooth tenderness, and no evidence of infection. She does have tenderness at the joints of her jaw. This is likely a TMJ syndrome (inflammation of the temporomandibular joint usually from grinding your teeth at night). It could also be impacted wisdom teeth. There is also the possibility of drug seeking. She is in no real distress, and is on a range of pain meds and psychotropic meds. Ding, ding, ding! Alarm bells here. Regardless, I'm not going to fix it here. I take a chance and I go ahead and give her a few pain pills with the recommendation that she check in with her dentist.

Three squads are inbound per the scanner. There are two MVA (motor vehicle accidents) victims, with one alleged ejection. There is also someone coming in by squad with back pain; Jesus, it just seems like a back pain kind of day today. Ejections are always very concerning because it usually means significant trauma.

In the meantime I see a 40-year-old white male who cut his right foot on a broken whiskey bottle at the local lakes. He was trying to get his boat out of the water. I see more of these kinds of injuries this time of year. There are way too many people not wearing shoes. We clean it and sew it up before the squad arrives.

There is also an 11-year-old white female who fell while skating at the local skating rink. She complains of left wrist pain. The films are okay. She goes with routine sprain instructions.

All righty, first victim. We have a 16-year-old white female restrained driver in the MVA. The person driving the oncoming vehicle in the other lane had fallen asleep at the wheel and crossed the centerline, sideswiping this patient's car. There is possible loss of consciousness, as the patient can't remember a period of time around the accident. She is on a backboard and has a cervical collar in place. Her primary complaints are her left thigh and right knee. Except for tenderness at these locations and some small facial cuts from a broken window, she is essentially unscathed. A key point though is that there was NO ejection, and only minimal traumatic injury. She is sent off for a range of films. We are scanning her head for good measure given this memory thing. We'll see...

Meanwhile, back at the ranch, we have a 15-year-old white male who sustained two small chin lacerations while wake boarding at the local lakes. One gets a few stitches and he's out the door.

The second victim arrives. This is a 16-year-old white female who was a restrained passenger in the same vehicle as the first. She complains of right knee and left upper arm pain and tenderness. I asked the squad guys about the other vehicle's occupants, and they tell me that that person refused transport. I send this girl off for some films.

The back pain turns out be a no show. They were either a no-transport or went the other way to an alternative hospital.

Meanwhile I see a 46-year-old white male with a cut on his right shin. It's hardly more than a nick, but he is sure it should be looked after. A Band-Aid is almost overkill on this injury. He's cleaned up and sent on his way.

Our second MVA victim comes back from X-ray first. All the films are fine. By this time she has found a couple of other spots, left forearm and hip, that hurt. So we send her back to X-ray for more radiation therapy. She's likely to have even more aches and pains come the morning.

Well we seem to be having a special on car wrecks. We have a demanding 43-year-old white female who comes in with her husband. They have just been T-boned (struck in the side) in their car. She wasn't wearing a seat belt and complains of right shoulder, right knee, and right lower leg pain. She also bopped her nose and had a transient nosebleed. There was no loss of consciousness, and her exam was benign. She is off to X-ray for some Medico-legal films.

In the meantime our second 16-year-old MVA victim is back for the second time. Everything is fine. She is sent home with her parents.

The first 16-year-old MVA victim becomes somewhat more complicated. She's had some vomiting and is feeling lightheaded. By this time her parents have arrived. I'm told that on several occasions in the past she has had memory lapses when she is stressed. She also has frequently vomited and fainted with blood draws, and minor surgical procedures. Oh joy. Essentially everything is normal on this kid except for some minimal cuts and bruises. We keep her for several hours, give her some fluids, and watch her. I give some significant consideration to keeping her overnight for good measure, but it all calms down, her support system is very reliable, and she wants to go home. I let her go.

Back to our 43 year old MVA. Everything is normal. She's out the door.

6:00 PM

Then it's back to (inappropriate) business as normal. We have a 21-year-old white male with a sore throat, achiness, cough, and fever for a few hours. He acts like he is dying. Of course everything is normal. Where do these people come from? He's got a viral syndrome, and I give him some symptomatic medicines.

Next is a 65-year-old white male with poison ivy rash for 4 days. He's going on vacation, and so of course it is a crisis today. I give him some Prednisone (a steroid) and some Atarax (an antihistamine). He's out the door.

The night is wearing on and the patients are queueing up fast.

We have a depressed looking 78-year-old white male who "just feels bad". The initial complaint is shortness of breath and cough. But then the real issue turns out to be his poorly controlled left sciatica pain. This is pain radiating down the back of the leg due to irritation or inflammation of the big nerve there. He was brought by a large group of family because they were concerned about the alleged shortness of breath. He had had a bypass several years ago and they "didn't want to take any chances." Now he was having no chest pain to speak of, and the shortness of breath was really more of a "I can't seem to take a deep breath." We do quite a work-up given the concerns, and don't really find anything. I treat him for a pre-sumed bronchitis, and more importantly, treat his sciatica more aggressively. He is scheduled to see his regular doctor on Monday.

Second is a frequent flyer. It's a 37-year-old white female with a day of nausea, vomiting, and abdominal cramping. She has a history of hepatitis, and is worried that it is returning. Of course, it's not. We give her some fluids and an anti-emetics, and send her on her way. She's feeling a lot bet-ter when she goes. It is more likely a routine stomach bug.

Third we see a 15-year-old obese white female with right ankle and knee pain. She fell while running after her dog. Her films are fine. She gets routine sprain instructions and is out the door.

Fourth is a 4-year-old white female who cut her right elbow on a bro-ken soap dish. I guess it didn't want to stop bleeding. It did need a couple of stitches. This little kid is actually a real trooper about it. She got quite a good haul of stickers, and went away happy.

Fifth is a 39-year-old white male with end stage diabetes. Looking through his old records, he had been non-compliant with his diabetic treatment since childhood, and is paying for it now. Small nerve injury associated with uncontrolled diabetes has given him a nonfunctioning bladder and he has a permanent catheter through his abdominal wall into his bladder. He's complaining of a week of intermittent lower abdominal pain. He's just tired of it and insists that he be admitted. Well the biggest thing that's wrong with him is that he is just packed with poop. Constipation is another common problem with diabetes, and he has it in spades. He might have a bit of a urinary tract infection as well, though he is on an antibiotic. We blast out the poop and give him a few days of a stronger antibiotic for good measure. He doesn't need hospitalization, and can follow-up with his regular doctor the first of the week.

Diabetes is a disease that is associated with a great deal of human suffering. It comes in two general flavors, Type I and Type II. In reality, there may be hundreds of different types, but for diagnosis and treatment at this time, it's easiest to consider this way. Type I, or Insulin Dependent Diabetes Mellitus (IDDM) usually occurs in childhood and is thought to be caused by an immune reaction that destroys insulin producing cells. These folks have an absolute lack of insulin, and must have it supplemented. Type II, or Adult Onset Diabetes Mellitus (AODM), usually occurs later in life and involves an acquired insensitivity to the body's own insulin. In these folks, if you actually measure insulin levels, it is usually elevated, but their tissues are not using it appropriately. This is usually managed with medicines aimed at increasing that insulin sensitivity, though there are a range of other approaches including giving additional insulin to overcome the insensitivity. The end result of both of these conditions, when uncontrolled, is elevated blood sugars.

Well, you might say, "so what?" The body doesn't like prolonged elevated blood sugars, and it can lead to a vast array of complications involving almost every organ system. These can be grouped into short term and long term complications. They can be further sub-grouped as to whether they affect Insulin Dependent Diabetics, Adult Onset Diabetics, or both.

Short-term complications in Insulin Dependent Diabetics can be catastrophic. If there is inadequate insulin, the blood sugar goes very high. This has an immediate effect on the kidney which spill the excess sugar into the urine, producing relative dehydration. Insulin is needed to get glucose, a primary nutrient for cells, into the cells. Without enough insulin, the cells begin to starve amidst plenty. They attempt to use alternate food sources, but this has the effect of increasing the acidity of the blood. As this spirals out of control, there is progressive vomiting, abdominal pain, lethargy, coma, and death. This progressive condition is known as diabetic ketoacidosis.

Short-term complications in adult onset diabetes are not so dramatic as with the insulin dependent diabetes. Since this is not a problem of an absolute lack of insulin, the cells don't starve, and thus the pathway producing increased acidity of the blood is not activated. The excess glucose does spill out in the urine, and can produce dehydration. As this progresses, it could reach the point where there is coma (called hyperosmolar coma), but this is uncommon.

Long term complication of Insulin Dependent and Adult Onset are very similar, they are also legion. Common complications include the "opathies". This includes neuropathy, nephropathy, and retinopathy.

Neuropathy is thought to be due to small vessel destruction in nerves that makes them malfunction. This produces characteristic (usually lower) extremity numbness and pain. It also leads to improper stomach emptying with recurrent vomiting, as well as abnormal intestinal motility with constipation. This is where you are also likely to get the atypical symptoms of angina in the diabetic; the small fibers of the heart that conduct pain are damaged, thus they get other symptoms like shortness of breath, rather than typical angina pain. Neuropathy can also lead to the bladder not functioning properly, as in this patient.

Nephropathy leads to eventual kidney failure, and may ultimately lead to dialysis. In fact the most common cause of renal failure requiring dialysis is diabetes.

Retinopathy leads to blindness. This occurs through a variety of mechanisms, but the outcome is the same.

Actually, the list goes on and on. Diabetes leads to vascular injury and early coronary artery disease. The persistent elevated blood sugar makes infection fighting cells less effective, and infection rates climb. And on, and on…

This doesn't even touch on the potential complications associated with diabetes management. Perhaps one of the most common is the diabetic reaction. This is where there is typically too much insulin for the glucose to be metabolized. It drives down serum glucose level and can lead to confusion, coma, and death. Lovely, huh?

So much for all of that. A bad, bad disease to have, but treatable. If treated aggressively, all of these complications can be avoided, or at least minimized. However, it requires a patient who is medically compliant for a lifetime.

Well, back to the rush of business. The sixth patient is a 25-year-old white female with sudden onset diffuse upper abdominal pain. It had been present 10 minutes, and was gone by the time I examine her. She had been having a lot of gas for the previous two days and is under a lot of stress. She does have a minor urinary tract infection, and may have either a little stomach bug or perhaps some stress related irritable bowel. It's hard to make too much of symptoms that are present for just a few minutes. She receives an antibiotic for the urinary infection and some symptomatic medicines. She can't have been in too much distress as she was laughing and joking pretty much from the moment she hit the door.

The night wears on, and seventh is an 11-month-old white female with low-grade fever, drooling, and decreased oral intake. She's got a lot of oral ulcers, and has the Hand Foot and Mouth Disease I have mentioned earlier. I give her some symptomatic medicines so she can take orals better.

The witching hour is approaching…

First though, my eighth patient in the rush, is a 43-year-old morbidly obese white female with low back pain since she was on a trampoline two weeks ago (and it's a crisis tonight). For whatever reason, something I am always attuned to is dental care, and this patient has perhaps three teeth in her mouth. We film her given the trauma aspect of the injury, and the fact that this is expected by the patient. Of course it's normal for age (after adjusting for the excessive weight). She's treated for a back sprain, and sent out the door.

The ninth and last patient of my shift is 51-year-old white female with a one week history of intermittent right frontal headache. This is similar to her prior "migraine" headaches. She's traveling, and didn't feel she could make the rest of the trip unless she could feel better. I made sure she felt better, and sent her on down the road. Her significant other was driving, so I imagine she slept through the trip.

Midnight and the relief crew is here. I am out of here, and not a moment too soon...

12:00 AM

Shift 6
"And what makes this a crisis tonight?"

Monday—18 Hours

12:00 AM

Another day in the trenches. We'll see how this one goes. It's hot and humid outside. The prior shift managed to get things cleared out prior to their departure. Yesss…

I get my schedule for next month. It's just what I asked for sweeeet…I wind up with just one overnight. How I manage that, God alone knows.

And we're off to the races. A 60-year-old white female who dropped a bench on her right foot has pain there. Films are fine. Ice, elevate, symptomatic meds and she's gone.

Next is a 4-year-old white male who was playing with his sister and somehow sustained a mid-forehead laceration. Both children are mum on just what happened. A little Dermabond (skin glue) and he is back together. For a painless 60 second procedure, this little guy sure puts up one hell of a fuss. Oh well…

I love my job. I love my job.

We've also got a 30-year-old white male, a truck driver, who complains of intermittent shakiness off and on for the past month. He chooses today and the emergency room to have it checked out. He smokes 2 packs of cigarettes a day and goes through 12 liter bottles of Mountain Dew a day. That alone would have me shaking to beat the band. He also relates that he has been under a lot of stress. He denies alcohol or drug use. Of course everything is going to be normal. I do some therapeutic testing just to appease the guy. We'll see.

On the scanner we've got a Code in progress at one of the local doctor's offices (someone has had a cardiac arrest). The squad is en-route. We start mobilizing folks to handle a cardiac resuscitation. I go and take a last minute pee, as who knows how long these things will go. Then the call comes through…, the patient has been stabilized and is going to be admitted directly. Yesss…Sometimes things just go my way. Unfortunately, that time is far and few between.

And as predicted, everything on our 30-year-old is normal. Looks like a combination of too much caffeine, nicotine, heat, stress and the like. He needs a lifestyle change, and I tell him as much.

The scanner has an unresponsive 74-year-old white female inbound by squad. Oh joy…

We simultaneously receive a call from the nurse of a local psychiatrist. They were sending in a person who may have taken an aspirin overdose. There is also a question of alcohol. She is reportedly lethargic. We'll see…

Well the alleged overdose is a bit more complicated than that. It's a 30-year-old white female who last night took perhaps 4 grams of Motrin (Ibuprofen). She's a bit cagey about this, but it was likely a suicidal gesture or suicidal attempt. It sounds like there are a lot of social issues involved where the patient may have to do jail time. Our job seems to be more medical clearance than anything else. She allegedly already has a bed at one of the local psychiatric facilities so we just have to clear her medically. We get started on drug levels and the like. Poison control is also contacted for their official recommendations.

Meanwhile we get the unresponsive 74-year-old white female. She had had a similar episode a couple of weeks previously, but no cause was ever uncovered. In fact she had a very detailed work-up that was pretty much normal. On exam she seems to be forcefully closing her eyes, and won't let you open them. There's nothing really localizing. We're obligated to rule out organic disease, but it really looks psychiatric. We'll see...

Another squad calls in. It seems to be someone with a recent hip replacement who had fallen and is having pain. The squad is ten minutes out and inbound.

Whoops, here she comes. Ten minutes is more like ten seconds. It's a 74-year-old white female I'd seen a couple of weeks ago who had split her femur around a prior hip prosthesis. It had since been repaired. She had had a NEAR fall today, and was having some pain. She wants the area X-rayed. Fine, we have the technology. Of course it was all fine. It takes more than a near fall to damage these prosthetics.

Back to our 30-year-old with the suicidal gesture. I'm able to clear her medically and send her on the way to the psychiatrists. These folks need a locked psychiatric unit that smaller hospitals rarely have. The local police, in our case, have a contract with a nearby community hospital to take care of these patients. If there is a life-threatening medical issue (as in an over-dose with something toxic) we hold on to them until they are medically stable, otherwise they are sent on their way. In this case our thirty-year-old goes by police cruiser. The police are better set up to handle potentially violent patients, and so this is the safest option for all involved.

Next is a 43-year-old white male who was using a hand held grinder at work. It kicked up and ground a chunk out of his nose. Luckily there was wasn't so much of a defect that it couldn't be closed directly. He is a bit of a wimp, with a capital "W", with the numbing though.

This is followed directly by a 40-year-old male with a huge scrotal abscess. This really isn't the immediate problem. Its been ongoing for a couple of weeks, and he's scheduled to have it drained in the morning. The real issue is that he was given Levaquin (an antibiotic) in the office today, and had some throat swelling almost immediately after taking it. These symptoms were almost completely resolved by presentation, so this is pretty much a no-brainer. I gave him a different antibiotic and an anti-histamine. He can follow-up in the morning as scheduled.

Then we have a 74-year-old white male with a history of known coronary artery disease. He had an angioplasty ten years ago, and hadn't had chest pain until now. He has been having chest pressure and shortness of breath through the afternoon. His EKG and lab are unchanged, but the patient is having angina until proven otherwise. Under ideal conditions angioplasty really only lasts about 7-10 years, so he's due. He is admitted quickly.

Then there is a 30-year-old white female who cut her leg canoeing several days ago. She is having increased warmth, redness, and pain at that site. It's obviously infected. I put her on dicloxacillin (a good antibiotic for skin infections) with follow-up.

Dinner time. The cafeteria has smothered burritos. They actually do a credible job at this.

It's an interesting thing about food and the Emergency Department. A great majority of ER's are essentially closed environments. Doctors, nurses, and techs go to work and usually cannot leave the area until their shift is over. There usually isn't any official lunch break, or really any break, period. Usually, the administration forbids reading magazines or such during down time; they don't want anything being done that the public might perceive as unprofessional. The long and short of it is that about the only thing you can do on the job that is at all enjoyable is eat. So there is always food around, and staff frequently have some degree of weight problem.

Well, back to it. Next is a 2-month-old white female who was sent over from her doctor's office for blood cultures and a dose of Rocephin (a broad-spectrum injected antibiotic). Why they can't do this over there I have no idea.

6:00 PM

I see a 65-year-old white male who had a skin cancer removed from his left forearm earlier in the day. He is complaining of tingling in the fingers of that hand. He has this huge dressing on the arm that is looped around each finger and is as tight as a drum. Just removing the dressing completely resolves the symptoms. We redress this tiny wound appropriately, and send him on his way.

Boy we are just stomping out disease and pestilence.

Then we have a 26-year-old white female who twisted her left foot and ankle 3 days ago. She just got off of work and wants it checked out. We do some therapeutic X-rays, and of course, it's just bruised.

The ankle is followed by a 27-year-old white male. He was kicked in the left face in his karate class, and managed an eyebrow laceration out of it. It's easily fixed with several sutures and he's on his way.

I've never understood it, but it seems that almost everyone who is getting sutures asks in advance how many it will take. I really wonder, what does it really matter? It's not like we're getting paid by the stitch. My usual response is "enough".

We then have one of our regulars, a 23-year-old white female with a migraine headache for two hours. She seems to be in about once a week or so. She's always very dramatic. Each time it's the worst headache ever. The real risk with these patients it that someday she may actually have something wrong, and we're likely to miss it. I give her my usual concoction and send her out the door.

Most Emergency physicians have one concoction or another that they use routinely for headaches. Whatever you do, you don't want to give narcotics. My experience has been that if you give narcotics you not only see that patient back more frequently, but you also see every other headache and pain patient who really needs some of that good Demerol (the most popular narcotic) for their excruciating pain. And of course nothing else will work for them…

Next is a 53-year-old Native American female with multiple pain complaints and recurrent vomiting. As is typical, she is an end stage diabetic. There is a huge amount of diabetes in the American Indian population. She has chronic neuropathic pain involving mostly her feet. She also has gastroparesis (a complication of diabetes that causes delayed stomach emptying) with chronic vomiting. Tonight she complains of headache, neck ache, back pain, chest pain, vomiting. She is very dramatic. This is likely a nothing in this patient, but we'll check it out. In the meantime we give her some IV fluids, Reglan (an anti-nausea medicine that helps with diabetic gastroparesis by increasing stomach motility) and some Toradol (a non-narcotic pain medicine).

Once again the squad is encoding. It's a 48-year-old woman with some kind of crush injury.

8:00 PM. It seems like I've been here a lot longer than that. Still 10 hours to go.

The squad arrives and it's a 48-year-old white female who allegedly crushed her right leg with her riding lawnmower. She shifted wrong and crushed it between the mower and what was reported as a fence. In reality it is a piece of heavy wire. The squad guys act like there was significant deformity of the leg and are sure there is a fracture. Again, in reality, there was a half-inch partial thickness cut that is hardly more than a scratch in the scheme of things. Sometime you just have to shake your head. The patient is discharged before the squad guys even finish their paperwork.

Next is a 6-year-old white male with a right sided ear ache for several hours. Both eardrums are blood red, which is definitely not normal. He's got an ear infection. Amoxicillin (an antibiotic) and Auralgan (a topical numbing ear drop) should fix him up just fine.

Next up is another regular, a 38 year old white female who's a long time alcoholic. She punched out a wall and is complaining of right hand pain and swelling. I've got to admit it looks like she has a boxers fracture (a fracture of the bone at the base of the small finger). Her films are fine though. She is just drunk as a skunk, and she just has a nice size hematoma (collection of blood under the skin) on that hand.

Well the witching hour is fast approaching and the craziness is beginning.

12:00 AM

The first patient is a complicated mess. It's a 13-year-old white female who had taken a swallow of a non-acetone based finger nail polish remover. It turns out this stuff was harmless. The real issue is whether this girl was trying to kill herself or just what. I know I'm in for a rough time when it is immediately apparent that she is 13 going on 30. I spend the better part of an hour trying to defuse and decipher the situation. Of course, all the while patients are building up in the lobby.

In the end, what was really going on is that she did this to get attention from her parents. She really wasn't trying to hurt herself. But the ground we had to cover was how she was sexually molested by a trusted third party when she was 10. There are huge issues surrounding this that are not going to be resolved in the emergency room. I really have to decide if this little girl should be committed or whether she is safe to go home with follow-up.

Of course the easy thing would be to commit her. Then she is out of my hair and become someone else's problem. It is my feeling with this girl that it would only make things worse. With all of this it doesn't help that I am a male. She might have related better to a female physician. I decide that there is adequate family support at home. Her parents will get her a psychiatric referral in the morning to get some help with her problems.

Now for the mess that's awaiting me. At least it's a bit easier. It's a 43-year-old white female who was knocked down by a horse that she was trying to train. She got a bloody nose out of it and some contusions and abrasions. We film her nose to ensure it was okay and it was. She is advised and released.

Then we have a 36-year-old white female, a road warrior, with back pain for years. It sounds like she had been in multiple car wrecks and received multiple beatings over the years and she looks it. She could easily have been 56. On X-ray Her spine sure looks like someone ten years older. I put her on some back sprain meds, and she was happy with that.

I'm being nickeled and dimed on these patients. I see a 21-year-old white female with one day of back pain. She is sure she has a urinary tract infection. She is also terrified that she might be pregnant. She does have a low-grade fever. The lab is normal, the pregnancy test negative, and so it is likely some type of viral syndrome. She wants to be on an antibiotic anyway, and I'm not really opposed. With some folks it just the path of least resistance.

This is followed by a 15-year-old white male with one day of left-sided abdominal pain and nausea. His exam is unremarkable, as is his lab. His belly films show quite a lot of gas and moderate stool. A thought had been a possible kidney stone, so we initially give him some IV fluids and Compazine (an anti-nausea medicine). With this minimal intervention his symptoms completely resolve. He likely has some combination of a viral stomach bug and constipation.

Next we have a 26-year-old white male with multiple tooth pain. He had been seen just the night before and injected with a local anesthetic, given pain pills, and referred to the dentist. The dentist allegedly wanted cash up front and he couldn't or wouldn't do this. It seems he is covered under another states Medicaid and so reimbursement is a problem.

Now patients like this I just don't understand. We are always joking about the patients who work at UNEM (unemployed) and see doctor NONE (these are entries in the cover sheet for employer and personal physician respectively). We are in the biggest economic boom in the history of the country, and here is this able bodied guy living on welfare, in other words you and me. I just don't understand it.

Well, of course, this guy wants pain meds. He tells me the Lorcet (a mild narcotic) is not strong enough. He does have really bad teeth, but it is questionable whether he is having the pain that he says he is. This guy sets off all sorts of alarm bells. He was in just the other night with another patient who was trying to get pain meds. When the nurse confronted him with this, he denies it, but there is no question he's the same guy. These folks somehow think we have a defective memory. He is a drug seeker in my book. I inject him again, but only concede a non-narcotic pain medicine. He's pretty upset about that, but tough.

Then we have a 57-year-old white female, another frequent flyer, with neck pain. She had just been seen in the office a few hours ago and diagnosed with a neck strain. She doesn't think the medicine she was given is adequate, and she just can't sleep. Well, neither can I. It's four in the morning, but rather than wait a couple of hours and see her regular doctor, we get to see her instead. I give her some non-narcotic pain medicine and send her on her way. She also is upset with this, but again tough.

Boy sometimes this job is frustrating. Next is a 20-year-old white female with several hours of a migraine headache. These occur when she has her periods. It hasn't responded to her home meds. Of course, she tells me that the only thing that works with her is Demerol. Not…I give her my usual concoction. It doesn't include Demerol, but if she truly has a migraine it will help, and it is that or nothing. I just refuse to give out narcotics on demand. She ultimately goes away.

The last case for my day is a twenty-year-old white male with one week history of intermittent mid-abdominal pain and vomiting. This is likely brown bottle flu. Of course he looks the part. He's also working at UNEM and a regular visitor of doctor NONE.

Six AM hits before the last case is half completed. A squad just arrived with an old woman with shortness of breath. I check out to the next shift, and I am out of here.

6:00 AM

Shift 7
"Talk about a shallow gene pool..."

Wednesday—18 Hours

6:00 PM

IIII'm back. Well back again.

There's one holdover and several in-processing. The holdover is a 79-year-old white male who came in chest pain. He is pain free at this time, and is waiting for his primary doctor to come in and admit him.

First business of the day, there are four patients, two parents and two children, who were in a MVA. They were all restrained. They were rear ended in their family car at a stoplight. There is minimal damage to the car. They drove to the emergency room and signed in 'to be checked'. Amongst them, there are no specific complaints. Their agenda is to have their necks "checked." I send them all en-mass to the X-ray department for cervical films.

One of the most important ways to minimize the complaints that makes administration so unhappy is to figure out the patient's agenda.

This is something I've talked about previously, and can really be a lot more difficult than it seems. Folks don't always let you know what they really want with any regularity. It is frequently dependent on their concept of appropriate medical care, and frequently has no resemblance to standard of care.

In this case the neck and the potential for neck injury was brought up on each patient. Since I have not yet perfected my X-ray vision, it makes sense that I just film these folks. Medico-legally you can justify it. It is also the path of least resistance.

All right, in the meantime I see a 46-year-old white male with a one week history of progressively more red and swollen left ear. He thinks a bug bit him. The ear is red, warm, slightly swollen, and tender. Looks like he's managed a local cellulitis, a diffuse skin infection involving the entire ear. I put him on some Keflex (an antibiotic effective against skin infections) and sent him on his way.

Okay, back to the MVA. We have a 37-year-old white male driver, a 33-year-old obese white female front passenger, a 13-year-old white male back seat passenger, and a 4-year-old white female back seat passenger. They all were restrained. There are minimal to no neck pain complaints with all of them. Of course their films are all normal. If anything, they all have some minimal neck sprains. Anti-inflammatories and tincture of time is the recommendation of the day. They are sent on their way.

All of this is followed by one of our regulars. It's a 35-year-old white female with a "migraine headache" for two hours. Surprisingly she came in under her own power rather than by squad as per her usual modus operandi; she historically calls 911. At least she takes whatever headache medicines I give her and goes away. Some time back she used to demand narcotics and refuse to leave if she didn't get what she asked for. I've previously had to threaten to have her physically removed by the local police when she refused to leave for want of Demerol. I give her Toradol, DHE, and Phenergan. These are a non-narcotic pain medicine, a migraine headache abortant, and an anti-nausea medicine respectively. Then, once again, she goes away.

I am so glad that we physicians as a group, here at this facility, rarely use narcotics for headaches and chronic recurrent pain syndromes. It has really cut down on the visits by the drug seekers. If they know they are NOT going to get what they want, they tend to go someplace else. That is A-okay with me.

Back to work. Next is a 65-year-old white female who cut her left index finger on a hedge clipper. A film is done to make sure the bone isn't involved, she gets four stitches, and is gone. Strong work!

This is followed immediately by a 25-year-old white male. He has cut his left index finger on a carpet knife. It's very superficial and does not involve any vital structures. Three stitches and he is done and gone.

Then we've got a 4-year-old white female with three or four days of nausea, occasional vomiting, diffuse abdominal pain. She's in no distress and her exam is normal. We'll do some lab and get a film of her belly. My impression is that this is likely a benign stomach virus.

Meanwhile I see a 15-year-old white male who was struck in the right elbow with a helmet at football practice. He also has a non-healing lesion of his right hand. His film is normal, so he's got a bruised elbow. With regards to his hand, he scrapped the hand a week ago, and has been dumping peroxide on it daily. He may as well have been dumping battery acid on it; daily peroxide can easily damage healing tissue. No wonder it's been taking a while to heal. I essentially told him, "Don't do that!" It's something of a no brainer.

And the race is on. I've got an 11-day-old white female with an emergency rash. She's also had a formula change today and had had some intermittent vomiting for the last 4-5 hours. Perhaps related, she's had very hard stools since birth. Her last stool was yesterday. She's had no fevers, but she has been fussier the last couple of days. She's been exposed to both Hand Foot and Mouth Disease, and to the stomach flu. On exam, she's got a large hard stool in her rectum. Given her age, I decide to get some lab and a film of her belly...

In the mean time I see a 32-year-old white female with a migraine since midnight. It was precipitated by the heat. She is a frequent flyer, usually with headaches. I gave her my headache cocktail minus the DHE because it is on her long list of "allergies." I think I've mentioned before how drug seekers are usually "allergic" to everything except their drug of choice, usually Demerol. She goes away.

Back to our 4-year-old belly pain. She has normal lab. Her belly-film shows a lot of gas and a lot of stool. There's no surprise here. On further exploration I find it's been 4-5 days since she pooped. Looks like she's constipated. She may have had a stomach bug as well. We'll get her cleaned out a bit, and otherwise treat her symptomatically.

Our constipated kid is followed by a 24-year-old Hispanic male with a sore throat and cough. Once again, hardly an emergency. He speaks no English and at least he brought along his English-speaking girlfriend. He's had a couple of days of fever, some sinus drainage, a sore throat, and a nonproductive cough. This is just the sort of stuff that you and I call a cold. Most importantly, he wants tomorrow off from work, and he needs a doctors note for this. I give him some symptomatic medicines, and his get out of jail card. "You deserve a break today..."

Then I see a 2-year-old white male with "bumps" on his head. His dad gave him a buzz cut, and they were just noticed tonight after the haircut. Uh, these are bug bites, and not exactly a crisis. Out of here...

Finally we've got something. I see a 2-year-old white male who ran into a door while playing. He complains of right shoulder pain and he's got a non-displaced clavicle fracture on that side. He gets a clavicle strap and some Lorcet elixir (a mild narcotic) for pain control. This will heal up just fine. He can follow-up in a week or so with his regular doctor.

Back to foolishness. I see a 15-year-old white male with right hip pain after football practice. He had planted his foot and twisted. He's essentially managed to sprain his hip. This is treated symptomatically, and oh yes, the instruction to not do that again.

12:00 AM

We've reached the Witching Hour…

And the fun never stops. I see a 23-year-old while male who was struck in the left temple with a frying pan a week ago by his girlfriend—some girlfriend. Given his appearance and demeanor, he probably deserved it. He has had a recurring headache since, and of course, it's an emergency now. A scan is done and normal, as is his exam. He's also apparently been under a lot of stress and hasn't been sleeping for more than a couple hours at a time over the last two weeks. This is likely as much the cause of his headache as the frying pan. He responds to headache medicine and is sent on his way. He needs to work on his stress management skills. I'm obviously not going to fix this tonight.

Then we're back to something real, a 10-year-old white male who had his tonsils out a week ago. He has been bleeding and spitting up blood for the last two hours. He's a keeper. These are scary things. I've seen way to many little kids holding large buckets of blood that they bled out in just a matter of minutes. It can rapidly be life threatening, and is very hard to control. About the only way to temporize this is to intubate these children and shove a pressure pack in the back of their throat. As you might imagine, that would be incredibly frightening to the child. Luckily the surgeon who had done the original surgery was on call, and he immediately took the child to surgery. Whew…

Back to the droll inappropriate Emergency Department visits, and a 41-year-old white male with one month of right sided back and leg pain. He had apparently done some lifting earlier in the day that made it worse. He had just had a MRI of his lumbar spine that showed some disk bulges, but nothing surgical. We got him comfortable, but he needs to follow-up.

Next is a 31-year-old white female with left neck pain for several days. This started after a Karate class where there had been a wide range of trauma. For the last day she has been noticing left shoulder weakness in addition to the pain. Cervical spine X-rays are done and are normal. There is still some concern of nerve impingement, possibly a cervical disk rupture. This is a medical urgency that warrants rapid follow-up. I offer to MRI her neck later in the morning when the machine is available, but she wants to follow-up with her regular doctor. An MRI is the study of choice to determine whether there is a problem in her neck that requires a surgical fix. It is possible to get these symptoms with a bad neck sprain and local inflammation, but it warrants the extra step to prove it. She seems reliable, and so it's reasonable to let her see her regular doctor in a few hours.

The bars are just closed so it's time for our 25-year-old black male frequent flyer. He's sure something is wrong with his arm. It's fine. He goes home. He is very drunk as usual.

Next is a 64-year-old white female with metastatic (widely spread) breast cancer who has multiple vague complaints. She's depressed and wants to be in the hospital. It is problematic whether I can find an adequate admission criterion. Though her disease is going to be fatal, it's not going to be fatal tonight. I'm unable to find anything that would pose an immediate threat or require that she be in the hospital. She's not real happy about it, but seems to understand what I have to say about it all. If she can't deal with life at home, she probably needs to consider a nursing home. She can talk with her regular doctor about this during regular hours.

This is followed by a 74-year-old white male with 30 minutes of right sided weakness. He has a history of hypertension, but has otherwise been healthy. He's never had a similar episode. Of course it is suspicious that he may be working on a stroke. His scan doesn't show an acute bleed, and his symptoms have been rapidly improving. He doesn't qualify for clot busting drugs, but has enough going on that it warrants admission for evaluation. I call his doctor and get him admitted.

Well we've been pretty much nonstop all night. It's now 5:00 AM, and the first time in 11 odd hours that the department has been empty. Now you know what my priority is don't you? Why sleep of course. My dictation can wait until later.

Zzzz...

6:00 AM

It wasn't much of a nap to speak of. It's 7:00 AM and time for the weekday morning clinic rush. This is folks who can't or won't see their regular doctor. Sometimes it's because they weren't able to get in a timely fashion. More often it's because it is inconvenient for them to have to wait in the doctor's office to be seen. They're stacking up quickly.

First is a 17-year-old white female who's had a sore throat for a week. She had gone to her regular doctor and had a negative strep screen and negative monospot. This means her sore throat was caused by something, usually a virus, that will not respond to antibiotics. She was put on an antibiotic despite the negative laboratory findings (current recommendations are to only give antibiotics to a strep positive sore throat). Well now, 5 days later, she has an antibiotic associated rash. At least her sore throat is better, but it would have been better in 6 days on an antibiotic or half a dozen days without one. We stop the Augmenten (an inappropriate antibiotic anyway), give her a dose of steroid, and put her on an antihistamine to get the rash under control. The moral of the story is that antibiotics have side effects, and they should only be used where they are likely to provide a benefit in excess of their risk of side effects.

Second is a 74-year-old white female with dizziness when she is upright. The dizziness precipitates nausea and vomiting. She has had multiple similar episodes in the past. Her exam is unremarkable. I give her some IV fluids, some Inapsine (a nausea/vertigo medicine), and some Antivert (a vertigo medicine). This makes her all better, and she goes home happy.

Third is a 19-year-old obese white female with sudden onset sharp left lower abdominal pain. She states that it "feels like gas." She's had no other signs or symptoms. She had a small hard stool this morning. Lab is all normal, and her abdominal films show lots of stool and lots of gas in her colon. We give her a Fleets enema, she poops and passes gas, and is cured. Ah, Emergency Medicine at it's finest, not.

Fourth we have a 33-year-old white male with a one hour history of palpitations and shortness of breath. Wow, this is potentially something real. He has a history of paroxysmal atrial fibrillation (an intermittent irregular heartbeat that can predispose a person to stroke, heart failure and the like). He is in atrial fibrillation now. I talk with his regular doctor and his cardiologist. I give him some Corvert (an antiarrhythmia drug), and he reverts back to a normal rhythm. He gets admitted for observation for the day.

Fifth is a 31-year-old white male with right ankle pain since last night. He twisted it when he caught his heel on a step. X-rays are normal, so he gets routine sprain care.

Sixth is a 30-year-old Hispanic male who had his left small finger crushed in a piece of equipment where he works. The film is fine. There is crush injury with a wound that is more of an avulsion laceration with maceration of the tissue. I pull it together with several stitches. He'll do fine.

Seventh is the 3-year-old white male child of a frequent flyer mother. He has allegedly had a cough for three weeks. He'd been on prednisone (a steroid) and a cough medicine. For the last several days to a week, he's had some green nasal drainage. I put him on Zithromax (an antibiotic). Given the alleged duration of these symptoms I can make an argument for a bacterial sinusitis. It would probably get better in time even with nothing, but the mother expects us to provide the cure.

Eighth is a 78-year-old white male with end stage supplemental oxygen dependent COPD (chronic obstructive lung disease). He was in the hospital a couple weeks ago with pneumonia. He relates that he just hasn't bounced back. He gets more short of breath with any exertion. He has essentially been little more than a lump for the past month, and is completely de-conditioned. Everything else is fine within the parameters of his known underlying disease. I offered a short Nursing Home stay with physical therapy, but he doesn't want that. He states that he will try and increase his activity gradually. I spend about 20-30 minutes talking with the patient and his family about what he needs to do to recover from this setback. They comment to the nurse prior to leaving that I had talked with them and told them more in my visit than their regular doctor ever has. This doesn't say much for some of the other doctors around.

This is a comment I get all the time. So many doctors, especially "old school" doctors don't really talk much with their patients or explain things to them. They seem to have an attitude of "do what I tell you, shut up, and don't ask questions." It's kind of sad.

Ninth, I see a 23-year-old white female, a patient of doctor NONE, who had some blood on her toilet paper after wiping. She has a couple of external hemorrhoids. After much discussion I find out that the real agenda is that her mother had a colon cancer at age 50, and she's worried about her risk for this. I refer her to a local doctor who can do an endoscopy. She can get a baseline sigmoidoscopy or colonoscopy to prove that her colon is normal.

12:00 PM

Well, it's now noon and I should be out of here. Unfortunately my relief called in and told me that he is going to be an hour or two late. I get the impression that he is in court and won't be done till then. Ah well, life is a bitch. I'll just keep plugging away…

The slate is clear, so I get to work on finishing up my dictations. No job's done till the paperwork's done, and Medicine has oh so much paperwork.

Lucky break, my relief broke all speed limits getting here and arrived just twenty minutes late. There are a couple of patients who have just checked in, but they aren't far enough along that they were ready to be

seen yet. It doesn't look like any of them have a problem requiring immediate attention. The incoming doctor leaped in and took over, and so I am
out of here...

Shift 8
"I am under-whelmed!"

Friday—18 Hours

12:00 AM

And we're off and running. There are no patients left over, but two new patients hit the door at about the same time as I arrive.

We have a 11-year-old white female who fell while running in the dark and injured her left lower leg. There's obvious deformity. X-ray shows a distal tibia fibula fracture. There isn't as much displacement or angulation of the fracture as you would expect given the appearance. I chat with the orthopedic surgeon, and we splint it for the weekend. She'll ice it, elevate it, and be on pain control and crutches till Monday. Then they'll likely cast it.

The other was an 18-year-old white male who was struck in the chest with a knee at football practice this afternoon. He's had increasing pain through the day. His films are fine. There's no sternum or rib fracture. Nor is there a pneumothorax (a collapsed lung). He'll be fine with symptomatic medicines. He's a bit of a wimp.

It's interesting to note that the biggest, most macho, guys tend to be the biggest wimps. In fact, men in general are wimps.

The classic is the buff dude with the huge tattoos all over his body who acts like you are trying to kill him when you give a tiny little tetanus shot. Talk about pathetic.

Back to my original train of thought. It's always a bad sign when you pull into the Emergency Room parking and see either multiple squads or multiple police cars. I've had occasion to pull in after 6-8 squads had just arrived. Needless to say, the outgoing MD is happy to see me on that occasion. Multiple squads usually mean trauma.

Police usually means a combative patient, a suicidal patient, or someone they had to forcibly subdue that needs medical clearance to go to jail. This later sometimes means that the alleged felon probably tripped several times getting into the squad car, if you know what I mean. Well...I guess to be honest, several of the local police occasionally just drop by because they want to chat for a while. Actually, they frequently have interesting stories to tell.

This brings up another interesting observation. The two groups of people who tend to be the most cynical are police and Emergency medical workers. We both tend to deal with the dregs of our society. We're routinely lied to, verbally abused, threatened, and the like. It's so much fun. It makes you really look forward to going to work.

Well things have slowed down as quickly as they started. I'm going to attempt some Zzzz's before the bars close.

Zzzz…

Well I managed about an hour. It's almost 2:00 AM so it's a given that there will be a rush.

I've got a 99-year-old white female from the Alzheimer's unit of one of the local nursing homes that fell and wound up with a left eyebrow laceration. Three sutures and back she goes.

Then a 73-year-old white male with foot pain for two weeks per the nurse. When I question him, it's more like a month. There's involvement of the base of the left great toe, as well as the adjacent toe. It is red, and slightly warmer. There's no demarcation. There are a lot of confounders. He has very bad vascular disease with significant venous stasis change. I did some general lab, but it's nonspecific. This could be chronic gout, but is more likely a neuropathic (nerve) pain due to his underlying vascular disease. He's on Coumadin and that really limits our medical options as it is incompatible with a range of medicines. It's very improbable that it's infection. We'll cover the gout angle with some prednisone and give him some pain pills. Given his age, I'll start with Darvocet N-100 (a Tylenol, propoxyphin [a mild narcotic] combination that's well tolerated by the elderly.) You really have to be careful with pain meds and old folks. Even Tylenol#3 (Tylenol with codeine) can make them real goofy. I've lost track of the folks brought in crazy as bedbugs from the relatively mild pain meds they were on. I've also lost track of the number of constipated old folks we've have to blast loose because the meds bound them up so much. Now prednisone isn't without its problems as well. Its side effect profile is as long as your arm, especially if taken long term. Short term, it can also make some folks a little weird, but this is a little less likely. Ah well, it's all a calculated risk/benefit equation. I'll have this guy follow-up first of the week.

My pillow is calling my name, but we get a call from someone who just can't pee. They're getting uncomfortable and want a foley catheter. This person should arrive in 20 minutes or so…or not. I'm going to get some rest. I'll deal with whatever happens when and if it happens.

Boy the scanner is alive with activity. The natives are restless. I'm sure it's likely to equate to more business. Again, I'll deal with it as it occurs.

Zzzz…

An hour and a half later and the 67-year-old white male who can't pee shows up; boy it sure was a long twenty minutes. He's had a problem with this for some time. It's due to an enlarged prostate. However, he's done fine since a microwave treatment at the first of the year. He gets a catheter and has something over a liter of urine in his bladder. There is no evidence of infection (it is sometimes a urinary tract infection that is the final straw that sets off these problems). He doesn't want to keep the catheter for the weekend. We remove it after his bladder is drained. We'll see him back as needed, and he can follow up with his urologist Monday.

Zzzz…

Next I have a 28-year-old obese white female who is very dramatic. She has a history of migraines and fibromyalgia, which right away fires up my radar that this visit could be primarily psychiatric. She complains of belly pain, migraine headache, right shoulder pain, neck pain, and passing out. We'll see, but my initial impression is that we'll not find anything. She seems awfully interested in what sort of pain medicine she might be getting. I order a range of studies and go back to bed.

Zzzz…

Well everything's back, and guess what, everything is normal with a capital "N." Hardly any surprise. Well she's a bit constipated and might have a borderline urinary tract infection, but nothing that accounts for these dramatic symptoms. I do some fancy talking, and convince her she's going to live after all. She's out of here.

One of our local police is here. He spent over an hour bull-shitting about this and that. He actually has a lot of good stories. Police have the same morbid sense of humor that Emergency Department personnel do. We all deal with the same death, destruction, and assorted low-life scum.

6:00 AM

Well the cafeteria isn't open weekend mornings. It's a vending machine breakfast. I found a Rueben sandwich and rounded up some Cappuccino from that machine. It fills the void.

That brings up another thing about Emergency Room work. You're essentially a captive in the hospital for the duration of your shift. About the only positive thing you're able to do for yourself is eat. As you might imagine, that makes it pretty easy to gain weight. What a lovely combination: sleep deprivation, limited physical activity, and lots of junk food. It shows in the nurses as well. There is almost always food on the counter, and literally everyone is carrying around extra pounds.

Well the natives are getting restless. They're waking up and have decided they need to be touched by a doctor. We've got someone coming in by squad and another was just wheeled into our trauma room. We'll see...

Okay an 88-year-old white female with recurrent episodes of chest pain at rest for the last 24 hours. She has known coronary artery disease. She has a left bundle branch block (an electrical conduction block that makes it impossible to decipher ischemia on EKG) that is unchanged. Her pain goes away with a single nitroglycerine. This is unstable angina until proven otherwise. She is a keeper, but we've got a bunch of stuff to do before we pass her off to the local docs.

The other patient is an 85-year-old white female with several minutes of general weakness while she was out for her morning walk. The symptoms are not localizing, she has no other specific symptoms, and she is symptom free by the time of presentation. Her exam was unremarkable. A TIA is improbable, but it could have been an arrhythmia. Her EKG is normal. Her lab is normal except for a full-blown urinary tract infection. She's also a bit orthostatic (Her blood pressure takes a drop between position changes from lying, sitting, and standing. This can reflect a range of things including dehydration, anemia, adrenal insufficiency and the like.) In this patient it would appear she is a bit dry. An antibiotic and some fluids should get her fixed right up.

A key aspect of Internal Medicine, the discipline associated with adult medicine, is the identification of typical problems that present atypically. This patients problem is a case in point. In a young person, a urinary tract infection will present as pain and burning with urination, urinary frequency and urinary urgency. In the elderly, none of these symptoms may be present. They often present with more nonspecific symptoms like weakness or confusion. Why this is the case is hard to say. I don't know that it is well understood. Though it is well documented.

Back to our chest pain lady. There is nothing to suggest that she is having a heart attack. I give her some protective medicines: an aspirin, oxygen, Lovenox (a blood thinner), Lopressor (a beta-blocker), and topical nitroglycerine (a blood vessel dilator). I then put a call in to her doctor, and she is whisked away into the bowels of the hospital.

In the mean time we have a 42-year-old white female complaining of right wrist pain. There is no definitive injury, but she said she heard it "pop" last night while she was engaged in normal activities. She is sure it is broken. How? We will do a therapeutic X-ray, because that's what she wants. She's another of these folks that are "allergic" to almost everything except the good stuff.

Surprise, surprise, the X-ray is normal. She's got a sprain, if anything. Of course she hadn't tried anything for it. I put her on standard treatment and sent her out the door.

Next is a 78-year-old white female who is worried that she has "pink eye". On exam she has had a small sub-conjunctival hemorrhage on the right. This is a big nothing. There is some bleeding under to conjunctiva of the eye. This is typically caused by a little broken capillary from rubbing the eye or the like.

I'm trying to work my way through a book on brain microstructure in my spare time this week. It's rather tough reading. In general though I'm having a hard time keeping my eyes open.

Zzzz…

12:00 PM

After a short nap I see a 17-year-old white male with right forearm pain since football practice yesterday. I just don't understand some of these kids. What? You figure you're going to spend days colliding with other kids and not have pain and bruising? His films are fine, the exam in pud. He's out of here.

We seem to be getting a steady trickle of patients.

We have a morbidly obese 39-year-old white female with a well-demarcated area of redness, warmth, and tenderness of her lateral ankle. There is no history of any specific trauma. It looks like a local cellulitis (an infection of the skin). It probably doesn't help that she must have a soap allergy. Why else would she look and smell like she hadn't had a bath in a couple of months? Boy, I just don't understand people. I put her on some dicloxacillin (an antibiotic with good activity against skin infections) and some naproxen (Aleve, an antiinflammatory). She should be much better in the next couple of days. I wish I could prescribe a bath.

Then we have a 1-month-old Hispanic child brought in because his belly seems "larger" to the mom, and he's not eating exactly on schedule. Can you believe this? The little guy is in no distress. He is pretty distended likely from swallowing a lot of air. The biggest concern is something the family isn't aware of and that is he has a fever. The child has a modest temperature and a significantly elevated white blood cell count. This demands a sepsis work-up in a child of this age. The child was admitted.

Children under the age of one month with a fever are at significant risk of certain bacterial infections. They are felt to not have a completely intact immune system, and studies have shown significant risk if fevers are not taken seriously. The work-up involves a chest X-ray, urinalysis, blood cultures, and spinal tap. They are then empirically put on intravenous antibiotics for a few days. As one would expect, the vast majority of these kids have nothing significantly wrong, but if it avoids one death for every fifty kids treated, it's still probably a reasonable investment.

Back to work. Next is a 70-year-old white female with intermittent upper abdominal pain yesterday and today. She has been under a lot of stress, and has a history of gallstones. The discomfort is cured with Rolaids taken at home, and she is symptom free at presentation. We'll check it out, but you have to wonder why she decided this should be evaluated in the Emergency Department.

Oh Joy, our frequent flyer, the 35-year-old white female with "migraine headache" from my last shift is back again. These folks get so old. They go to the Emergency Room again and again with their chronic non-emergent complaints. These folks rarely follow-up during regular hours. I give her my concoction, and encourage her to see her neurologist on Monday. Who knows?

Next in our cavalcade of walking well is a 24-year-old white male with a week of fever, sore throat, swollen glands, and fatigue. I do a Strep Screen and a Monospot, and the Monospot is positive. This kid has mononucleosis (the mono you always hear about). It sounds like his girl-friend may have the same bug. It's a viral illness caused by the Epstein Barr virus. There is no cure, just symptomatic treatment. The usual recommendation is plenty of fluids, Tylenol, and the like. They can have symptoms for as long as six to eight weeks, so it is something of a drag.

In our asymptomatic 70-year-old with the transient abdominal pain, all the lab and whatnot is normal. This is likely a case of acid reflux secondary to anxiety. She could have some biliary colic as well, but this is not supported by ultrasound. I think it is very low probability that this could be cardiac, which is something you always have to think about in these patients. Well anyway, everything was normal. I suggested she restart her Prilosec (a medicine that turns off stomach acid production) and follow-up the first of the week.

The end of my shift is in sight. Only one and a half hours to go.

We've got a 77-year-old white male who tripped at home this morning and now has right lateral foot pain. He's managed to fracture his proximal fifth metatarsal. This is the bone that the small toe attaches to. We treat this with a post-operative shoe (a wooden soled shoe), crutches, and partial weight bearing. He'll be seen again in a few days by the orthopedic surgeon.

An hour and counting. Little old clock-watcher me. Hey, for a weekend shift it's really been pretty pud.

The relief crew is in and I am out of here…

6:00 PM

Shift 9
"My fun meter is pegged!"

Monday—18 Hours

6:00 AM

I scared the hell out of the prior shift's doc when I woke him to take the baton. It couldn't have been that bad of a night if he was sleeping that soundly.

Wouldn't you know it there hadn't been a patient since 3:00 AM, I'm not here 60 seconds, and someone is beeped in.

All right, my first crisis is a 26-year-old white female who is a couple of weeks out from a spontaneous vaginal delivery. She has had intermittent cramping and spotting since the delivery that is worse this morning. Of course she hasn't discussed this with her obstetrician prior to presenting to my Emergency Room. Now the real agenda is that earlier in the week an on-call gynecologist had mentioned that there could possibly be retained placenta, and that they might have to do an ultrasound and a D&C. So she's decided that now is the time to have an ultrasound. It makes no never mind that the doctors offices open in an hour and a half, and that even if there are positive findings that nothing would be done for this before the afternoon, at the earliest. Ah well…Service with a smile. I order her the ultrasound as well as some varied laboratory tests.

Meanwhile we have a 27-year-old white male with a five day history of pain at the base of the right great toe. He has no doctor, and has made no effort to obtain one, so it becomes our problem. There is no history of trauma. There is a slight amount of redness and significant tenderness in the area he is concerned about. I order lab and an X-ray. Gout is a possibility, though he's a bit young for it.

Well, it's a bit after 7:00 and patients are starting to stack up. This is a typical Monday, clinic, clinic, clinic.

Third is a 55-year-old white female with upper abdominal pain through the night. She has a known history of gallstones, and she does have focal right upper quadrant tenderness that would be consistent with gall bladder disease. We'll see what we have.

Fourth is a 79-year-old white female with two months of exertional shortness of breath. It's no worse today. She just can't wait until her Friday appointment, though she has made no attempt to have it moved up. She seems like a real Nervous Nelly. Her vitals are normal, as is her exam. We'll do the cardiopulmonary work-up and see if we find anything. My initial impression, especially given her demeanor as well as her repeated comments about being alone, is that he may have problems with depression and anxiety. We'll see...

Our 26-year-old with the cramping and vaginal spotting had normal lab and an unremarkable ultrasound. The scan was just consistent with a post-partum state. After discussion with the same on-call gynecologist she had talked with previously, we put her on methergine (a uterine contracting medicine). She can follow-up later today for a recheck. If she doesn't respond to the methergine she may need a D&C, but it won't be today.

Our 27-year-old guy with the big toe pain probably does have gout (a uric acid metabolism problem that leads to uric acid crystals in joints, and subsequent pain). His uric acid level is through the ceiling. I put him on some Indocin (an anti-inflammatory that is very effective in gout) and Tylenol #3. He needs to follow-up with a local doctor.

Something over 50% of folks with a flare of gout will have a recurrence in a year or less. Some folks need to be on allopurinol, a medicine to chronically suppress the formation of the crystals. This isn't something I'm going to start out of the Emergency Department.

Back to our 55-year-old with belly pain. She's all better with some Compazine (an anti-nausea) and Toradol (an anti-inflammatory). Her lab is fine, but her belly films show marble sized gallstones. I decide to get an ultrasound to see if it's inflamed. Then the plot thickens.

This lady's had intermittent pain for years. She doesn't want to even consider having her gallbladder out until her insurance kicks in three months. She's been trying to hold out until then.

Well the ultrasound is completed and shows the stones, but no evidence of significant inflammation. It looks like she can try to baby this along for a few more months.

The scanner has a 53-year-old white male coming in with a migraine headache. Oh joy…

Back to our 79-year-old with the shortness of breath. She does have a history of congestive heart failure, and had been on blood pressure medicines that are also used to treat heart failure. These were discontinued about the time her symptoms started. Her weight is up over five pounds to a beefy 95 pounds. Her chest X-ray does show some mild failure, but she is not hypoxic. She has no other findings. I give her a dose of Lasix (a diuretic) and restart her meds. This is coordinated with her regular doctor. He indicates that it was an oversight that all the medicines were discontinued. She had been having problems with low blood pressure at the time, adjustments were made, and she was lost to follow-up. He concurs with my intervention and will see her in a couple of days for a recheck. I guess it wasn't depression and anxiety after all, although these likely played some role here.

Well our 53-year-old white male showed up. He's got a history of migraine headache, and this is typical for him. It's throbbing, with nausea, vomiting, and photophobia (light sensitivity). Of course his exam in unremarkable, except for an Oscar winning performance for best dramatic acting. I'll give him my usual concoction, and we'll see how he does.

In the mean time I see a 22-year-old white female with a painful swelling in her left armpit for a week. Of course it's a crisis today, and she can't wait until her appointment tomorrow to be seen. She's got a little infected sweat gland. By her dramatics you would think she was going to die from this. I went ahead and drained it (a chore in and of itself) and packed it. I put her on an antibiotic, and a pain med. She is out the door. She can keep her appointment tomorrow to have the packing pulled and changed as appropriate.

In the meantime, our 53-year-old dramatic male headache patient has gotten a second round of headache medicines. He was about 50% better, but isn't quite good enough. He's a bit dizzy with the meds. We'll watch him a while longer. If this doesn't take him pretty much to baseline, I think we'll scan his head.

I receive a call from Cardiac Rehabilitation about a female cardiac patient who developed an arrhythmia. They are bringing her on down.

In the meantime we've got a 37-year-old white male who was struck in the left ear with the edge of a cabinet. He's got a nice ear laceration. Six sutures and he is gone.

This was followed by a 23-month-old white female. She had fallen from a shopping cart at a local department store. There was no loss of consciousness, and she's been appropriate since. She has a small scalp wound that when cleaned, is little more than a scratch. There are no other injuries. A dab of Neosporin, a head sheet, a wound sheet, and she is gone.

The lady from cardiac rehab is 73 with a history of atrial fibrillation. She was shocked back into a normal rhythm about a month ago, and had just been given a clean bill of health. Today she's back in atrial fibrillation. Her rate is fine and she is having no symptoms. I coordinated with her cardiologist. We put her back on Coumadin and Lovenox (blood thinners) to reduce stroke risk, and she'll follow-up later this week.

Then we're back on of my favorite past-times, road warriors! Not. I see a 40-year-old white male who drove a large nail through his hand with a pneumatic nailer. He missed everything vital. I numb it with Lidocaine (the novacaine that dentists use), and pull it out with my fingers. He needs to follow-up later in the week for a recheck. Who knows if he will?

This is followed immediately by a 30-year-old white male with a scratch on his left index finger. He wants a tetanus booster, and just does-n't want to wait till tomorrow.

Sounds like there's a little old grandma coming over from a local nursing home with a possible hip fracture. We'll see...

The squad is out to one of the local restaurants for an older lady who twisted her ankle. Oh joy...

The nursing home grandma is a 88-year-old white female who slipped out of her wheel chair and landed on her butt. I send her off to X-ray, and the answer is...left pubic ramus fracture. This is a stable fracture of one of the bones in the pelvis that you sit on. It's treated with pain control and heals on its own in 6 to 8 weeks. She's going back to the nursing home.

Oh lovely, a three beeper from the triage area. This means cardiac or respiratory case usually.

...And it's an 88-year-old white male who has been sweating today and is sure he's having some severe medical problem. He has no other symptoms. Now, there's something about it being 99 degrees and 99% humidity outside that may contribute to this. The gentleman is acting like has is suffering an absolute lack of Xanax (a tranquilizer). He also comments that he is out here to the Emergency Department "all the time" and that we "never find anything." This says something, doesn't it?

We've also got a 23-year-old white female who's six weeks pregnant with vaginal spotting. She has an appointment to see her regular doctor this afternoon, but would rather come here. An ultrasound done a week ago didn't look good, but the quantitative HCG (a measure of fetal viability) was still rising. Her agenda is that she really wants a repeat ultrasound. Of course you know our motto, "have it your way...".

Finally we get the 70-year-old white female in by squad with left ankle pain. She missed a curb at a local restaurant. She hadn't tried bearing weight before being brought in. Her films are normal, and when we stand her, surprise, she is weight bearing with no difficulty and very little pain. Well what do ya know?

The day is dragging on. At the tone, the time will be 3:00 PM.

I see a 24-year-old white male with one week of an itchy rash. He's got a contact dermatitis, like poison ivy, poison oak, or the like. Some steroids and an antihistamine and he'll be better quicker.

Our 88-year-old sweating male is all-normal except for a low thyroid function. He is on thyroid replacement and is likely not taking it. His regular doctor had checked the level just a few weeks ago and it was therapeutic. In talking with this doctor, it sounds like this has really been a problem patient with recurrent medical noncompliance issues. I reassure the patient that he's going to be fine. He seems happy that we found something, but doesn't' make the connection that it is really his fault for not taking his medicine. I arrange follow-up with his regular doctor later in the week.

The 23-year-old pregnant girl with the spotting is having a miscarriage. Lab and ultrasound don't look good.

In excess of ten percent of all first trimester pregnancies end in miscarriage. People really need to be reassured that it is nothing that they did or didn't do. They also really need to know that it has little bearing on future pregnancies.

This patient will follow-up with her regular doctor later this afternoon as scheduled.

12:00 PM

Food, food, food. I sometimes feel I have little else to look forward to when I'm at work. Barbecue beef and beans. At least it's palatable.

Hmmm. There seems to be a bit of a lull. I've been finishing up my dictations and trying to do a bit of reading. I'm sure it's not likely to last long.

Read, read, read…

Well we managed two whole hours of relative peace.

Now we've got a completely noncompliant insulin dependant diabetic to cope with. It's a 28-year-old white male who complains of shortness of breath with exertion and at rest for the past five weeks. He essentially states that he has no insurance, no money, and that it is our responsibility to provide a course of treatment to cure his current condition. This is definitely a no win situation.

The Emergency Room is not really set up to provide end-to-end medical treatment to the indigent. Years ago pharmaceutical reps would stock medicine samples. This would allow medicines for those folks who couldn't afford them. That practice has fallen by the wayside for whatever reason. Hospital policy doesn't allow dispensing any more medicine than is needed to get the patient to the pharmacy when it's open next. They don't want to get stuck with the additional expense of medicines. It is frustrating to deal with patients like this. They have enough money to buy cigarettes, but not enough to buy even inexpensive medicines.

What am I going to do with this guy? I'll treat him like any other patient regardless of ability to pay. So many of these folks know the system and try to manipulate it to their best advantage.

A real problem, too, is that these folks often have real and severe medical problems. If you treat them any different than any similar patient, or miss anything, I guarantee you they know the phone numbers of a ambulance chasing lawyer.

So, in the end, this person's self abuse and medical noncompliance becomes my problem rather than his own.

I do the work-up and what did I tell you, this guy has a big pneumonia. It's not bad enough to make him hypoxic, but it's going to get worse if not treated adequately. Social Services doesn't have any help for an otherwise able bodied 28-year-old male, and I'm sure he will not fill a prescription if

I just give him one. I'm faced with either bringing him in daily for 10-14 days for an injected antibiotic or brow beating pharmacy into attaching an oral antibiotic course to the bill he's not going to pay anyway. Since it's going to cost the hospital either way, I think pharmacy is going to buy off on it.

I manage to get this guy an entire course of antibiotic plus breathing medicines. Of course there's no thanks from this guy that I just brow beat $200 worth of medicine out of the pharmacist. I just shake my head.

6:00 PM

Let's move on to the next patient. We have a 5-year-old Hispanic male who is hysterical. He has a twenty-minute history of belly pain and nausea. His exam is unremarkable except for his wailing and carrying on. I'm betting he just has a stomach bug, or maybe he's just constipated. He has had some small hard stools. We'll check it out.

In the meantime we have a 2-year-old white male who got sand in his right eye at day care. And boy do we dig out some sand. Remarkably, there was no corneal injury. I put him on some antibiotic eye drops for good measure.

Our little Hispanic boy was cured with a Phenergan suppository (an antinausea medicine). His lab is normal and his belly film just shows lots of gas. Looks like he's got a little stomach bug. We'll treat this symptomatically for now.

Next is a 53-year-old white female who smokes 2 packs a day. She's had cough and cold symptoms for 3 days, and complains that she get these symptoms frequently. She doesn't seem able to make any association between her heavy smoking and her recurrent respiratory illnesses—go figure. This is the power of denial at work. I get her a cold pack (antibiotic, antihistamine, cough medicine) and send her on the way. This is likely a viral illness exacerbated by her smoking-induced chronic bronchitis, but folks like this expect to walk out with the cure.

Well the winners are back out in force. We've got a 25-year-old white male with an alleged migraine headache. Of course he makes sure I'm aware that all of the routine headache medicines don't work on him.

I've also got a 30-year-old white male who punched out a wall with his left hand. Now this is the work of a real rocket scientist. We'll see what the film shows. And the answer is…normal. He's got a nice hematoma (a collection of blood under the skin). He deserves the pain, but I'm a nice guy so I give him some Tylenol #3. Ice, elevate, and don't do such stupid stuff again.

Midnight is coming up but nowhere near fast enough…

Midnight's here and I'm out of here.

12:00 AM

Shift 10
"Take deep breaths, and walk towards the light…(Thanks, Monte)"

Wednesday—18 Hours

12:00 PM

Well we're off to a racing start right out of the chute. There was no one here when I arrived, but multiple people checked in promptly at noon. But it's a clinic, right?

First is a 27-year-old Hispanic male with a three day history of sore throat, left ear pain, and left ear drainage. Of course he has no doctor. He's got an external otitis as well as an otitis media on the left (infection both in the ear canal as well as behind the eardrum). Treating this will treat a strep infection if he happens to have strep throat, so I don't even check. I put him on Amoxicillin (an antibiotic) and Cortisporin (an antibiotic/antifungal/steroid ear drop) and sent him out the door.

I've also got an 8-month-old white female who had gotten a foot caught in a shopping cart at one of the local stores. This seems to be a frequent problem these days. It required the cart to be cut away from the foot at the store. There is no obvious injury, but the family is here to have it filmed, so we'll do what they want.

We've also got one of our headache regulars, a 24-year-old white female with a "migraine headache." She's been in a half dozen times in the last week alone.

To top it all off we have a squad inbound with a 10-year-old who had a seizure.

The shopping cart kids X-rays are fine. She just has a bruised ankle. Tylenol or Motrin is all that's needed, if anything.

Our headache person and her husband are telling me that they are going to a specialty headache clinic. They just want "something to help her travel." I give her the benefit of the doubt, but somehow I don't think this new clinic is going to cure her. A large percentage of her problem is psychiatric. Who knows though, maybe this clinic is clued into the psychiatric component of a lot of these patients.

The seizure patient finally arrives. It's a 10-year-old white female who had had a couple of headaches earlier in the week. Last night she had a headache, decreased vision, and some confusion. She was seen at a regional Emergency Department and a complete work-up was done that failed to show any specific pathology. Her symptoms were attributed to migraine headache, she received a migraine medicine, and got much better. Today she had a one minute episode of shaking, and was a little confused afterward. It sounds a bit like a seizure, though it's a bit atypical. She has no prior history of seizure.

This child is pretty much baseline by the time I examined her. There's no specific physical findings at this time. I start some basic lab, and send for records from the hospital she were she had been evaluated.

In the meantime I see a 79-year-old white male with three hours of left-sided weakness and numbness. He has a history of multiple strokes, and was just in the hospital a couple of weeks ago after his most recent episode. I start the work-up.

With our 10-year-old I verified the work done at the other hospital. We did find a urinary tract infection that we began treating, but it is unlikely that this is related to her current symptoms. With a negative work-up as performed, the likelihood of something threatening is minimal. I chat with her regular doctor and he will arrange for neurology referral.

Our 79-year-old with the weakness and numbness has a normal lab and unchanged head scan. He'd had a complete work-up just last month looking for treatable causes of stroke that had no significant findings. Well, he's obviously failing his current therapy, so he's admitted. Perhaps the neurologist can come up with a plan.

We have a slight lull.

Next I see a 9-year-old white male who jammed his left small finger at school. He's got a small fracture, but it's well aligned. I splinted it and arrange for orthopedic follow-up. They apparently have both a regular doctor and an orthopedic doctor and, for whatever reason, are not happy with either of them, hence they showed up here.

Then I see a 10-year-old white male who twisted his right ankle at school. He has pain in his right lateral ankle, but the X-ray is normal. We'll treat with routine sprain instructions.

This is followed by a 27-year-old white male who twisted this right knee 3 days ago. He works at UNEM and sees doctor NONE. Of course the films are normal. Ditto on the sprain instructions.

Boy I'm just having loads of fun. I see a 34-year-old white female, very dramatic, complaining of a "migraine headache." She is sent over from her regular doctor's office "to get a shot." We received no call from this doctor, and of course she says that nothing works better than Demerol. No doubt…But, I think not. I give her my routine concoctions, and she has to settle for that.

Then a 56-year-old Hispanic male, a patient of doctor NONE. He's been on Hytrin (a blood pressure medicine that also helps folks with an enlarged prostate gland) for his enlarged prostate. He was put on this when he was in Mexico. He ran out a couple weeks ago and is having a more difficult time urinating. These are typical symptoms of prostate hypertrophy. I need to verify that he doesn't have a urinary infection before I put him back on the Hytrin.

Then yet another patient of doctor NONE, a 25-year-old white male with cold symptoms. I think he really wants a get out of jail free card so he doesn't have to work tonight. Of course we want to keep our customers happy. Sometimes I think we should just leave blank signed forms in the lobby.

My 34-year-old headache lady received Nubain, Vistaril, Reglan, and Thorazine. At last she's ready to go home. We took her headache from a 10+ to a 1 without using Demerol. I must say I am surprised. She's poured into her car, and her husband drives her home to put her to bed.

Our Hispanic with the peeing problem is also a diabetic. We find this on the urinalysis. This is something he neglected to mention. It seems he only takes his medicine when he thinks about it. Also, it turns out that it has been 4 months since he has had his prostate medicine. I put him back on the Hytrin at bedtime and recommended he take his Glyburide (a diabetes medicine) at the same time so he's less likely to forget it. Then I impress upon him that he needs a local doctor real soon. I only give him enough Hytrin for a couple of weeks, so this should make it more likely that he complies with the follow-up request.

Oh boy, now for a "real" emergencies. It's a 27-year-old white male with a sebaceous cyst for which he wants an antibiotic. He also complains of anxiety and recurrent headache. He wants some Xanax (a tranquilizer) and a pain medicine. Once again it's doctor NONE. I give him a few of what he wanted, but tell him that anything further will have to come from a primary care doctor.

6:00 PM

Next is a 10-year-old white female who fell from her bicycle while racing a friend. There was no loss of consciousness. She's got a small goose egg. There are no other injuries. Her parents brought her in because, "it swelled up so fast." They act like she is about to die. I just don't understand people like this. I don't think I'd bring in my child for something like this. It's noteworthy that, of course, she wasn't wearing a helmet. She'd have no injuries at all if she had been wearing recommended protective gear.

Next we have a 30-year-old white male who cut the web-space of his right thumb and index finger with a utility knife. It isn't deep enough to do any real serious damage. I put three stitches in it and send him on his way.

Then there is a 10-year-old white male who had his bell rung in football practice this morning. He's had some nausea and intermittent dry heaves since. He likely has a mild concussion despite no loss of consciousness. We'll scan his head to prove there's no bleed or fracture, and then we'll treat him symptomatically.

Hmmm. Bicycle injuries abound today. Next is a 46-year-old white female who fell off her bicycle. She's got a chin laceration and some wrist pain. The X-rays are fine, but her chin requires some suturing.

We also have a 20-year-old white male, yet another patient of doctor NONE. He complains of emergency jock itch, anal itch, athlete's foot, painful urination, sore throat, and ringworm.

We've also got his 21-year-old girlfriend. She thinks she may be as much as 4 months pregnant. She's got a history of a kidney stone and has a stint there that was supposed to be removed some time ago, but she was lost to follow-up. She's been having blood in her urine and discomfort with urination. She's also voiced some concern about sexually transmitted disease. Both of these kids are able bodied and unemployed. I start some lab to better figure things out.

In the meantime I see a 14-year-old white male who put a nail through his tennis shoe into his left foot. These injuries have a high incidence of infection with an unusual organism known as Pseudomonas. Because of this, we'll cover him with an antibiotic after we prove there is no injury to the bone and that no shoe material is in the wound.

Back to our 20-year-old male with the myriad complaints. He's got a lot of fungal rash that could have easily been cured with an over the counter preparation like Lotrimin. He's got a viral sore throat. He doesn't have a urinary tract infection, so it makes one wonder about gonorrhea or chlamydia. He vigorously denies that he is as risk for either of these, but I talk him into checking just the same. However, I can't talk him into empiric treatment. He'll call back for results.

Lovely, a squad is inbound with a 30-year-old white male who fell off his bike.

Our 21-year-old female is pregnant. Her urinalysis looks like crap. I did an ultrasound as well, and we're still waiting for the results.

And what do you know, the squad brings in a 30-year-old drunk bicycle rider. He was so drunk that he couldn't stay on his bike, and just fell off. He's got a small superficial abrasion of his left eyebrow, but otherwise no specific complaints. His exam is fine. He's out of here with a head sheet, wound sheet, and follow-up as necessary.

Boy, the drunks just keep on coming! We've got another 30-year-old white male with mid-abdominal pain for the last couple of days. He drinks a 6 to 12 pack a day. He's tried all the over the counter meds without much improvement. Surprise, surprise he routinely sees doctor NONE.

Both our 20-year-old and a 21-year-old tell me that they have no money to spend on medicine, and so they are not going to get their scripts filled. They have money for cigarettes,…oh why do I even bother? Well his jock itch isn't likely to kill him. Her kidney infection could. I gave her a dose of antibiotic tonight, and recommended she follow-up with the urologist tomorrow. I'm sure he could give her medicine samples from his office, if she bothers to follow-up appropriately. And to think that these idiots are going to have a child, pity the child.

9:00 PM

Folks are still queuing up.

I see a 2-year-old white male who put the plastic eye of a stuffed animal in his ear. It is right there and easily removed with an alligator forceps.

Back to our 30-year-old with belly pain. He has a world class case of pancreatitis (inflammation of the pancreas). Surprise, surprise. This is a condition that can be life threatening. It warrants hospitalization. He had 50mg of intravenous Demerol and it hardly took the edge off his pain. There are multiple potential complications of this disorder, many of which can easily end in death. And wouldn't you know it, this guy doesn't want to be in the hospital. This is really typical of hard core alcoholics. They are frequently worried that they will go into withdrawal or have the DTs (delirium tremens) if they go without the alcohol. Despite using the death word multiple times, he would not be swayed, and he left against medical advice. Ah well, you can lead a horse to water, and all that…On to more important things.

Zzzz…

12:00 AM

Surprise, surprise. Heeeee's back. Our pancreatitis guy only lasted 2 hours at home. He's quickly admitted.

Zzzz…

I'm awakened to a 20-year-old white man who cut his left thumb on a piece of metal at work. It's just barely deep enough to need stitches. You would have thought I was killing him when I was repairing the wound. Men are such wimps. Ah, well he's out of here.

Zzzz…

4:00 AM

The next crisis I'm awakened to is a 2-year-old white male with no bowel movement in 2 days. He was apparently more fussy for the last day. The family members just "didn't know what to do." How about call your doctor, or have him checked out in clinic during regular office hours. The child is in no distress and immediately poops after the digital stimulation of a rectal exam.

Well it must be a full moon. We've got a 22 year old white female who complains of a half hour of confusion, some transient right face and hand tingling which has since resolved. Since she arrived, she complains of a mild all over headache, similar to prior headache. This girl just seems nuts…My initial impression is to ask what is she on? She does have a history of pseudotumor cerebri a couple of years ago. This is a condition that leads to recurrent headache. We'll do the big neurological work-up. In addition I'll do a drug screen. Somehow I don't think I'll find anything.

I also hear on the scanner that the squad is out to one of the local old people places. Oh joy…Almost immediately, the squad encodes and it's an 87-year-old white female who had taken a fall.

We're close to 6:00 AM and where is my relief crew? I'm anxious to get gone, so he can figure out this crazy woman. He's here. These folks are his, and I am out of here.

6:00 AM

Shift 11
"There's badness going on!"

Friday—18 Hours

12:00 AM

I'm beat. What a way to start a weekend. I'm told it's been continuous all day; the natives are restless. It's hot and humid outside, just the thing for the lungers to come running on in. It just feels like a full moon.

Zzzz...

Well I tried to get a bit of rest, but I guess there's no rest for the wicked. I've got an 80-year-old white male with 2 hour history of chest pain with radiation into both arms. His EKG is nonspecific, and he has no significant medical history or risk factors aside from advanced age.

I've also got a 21-year-old white female with a heavy period and cramping. It's been going on 24 hours and is a crisis now. It's not any worse, just hasn't gotten better.

There's also a squad out for someone with chest pain and shortness of breath. Oh joy.

I also hear the police on the scanner with a juvenile they are bringing in to have something checked.

...And we've got folks in the lobby checking in.

The squad is a 39-year-old white female with sudden onset upper abdominal pain. This is a patient with a history of multiple abdominal surgeries, and she's also got quite a psychiatric history. It's such a lovely combination. Combine this with a severe dose of dramatics and it all makes for a zoo.

Our 80-year-old received routine cardiac meds (aspirin, oxygen, beta-blockers, heparin, and nitrates) with pretty much complete cessation of his pain. The kicker is that the second EKG shows a new anterior-septal myocardial infarction in progress. I chat with the on-call doctor, and we will hold TPA given that he's symptom free. He's up to the ICU.

And this is quickly replaced with a 29-year-old white male with sudden onset left flank pain. He's got blood in his urine, and likely has a kidney stone. I arrange an IVP.

I've also got a 21-year-old white female with painful right ear for 6 months. Just had taken out an earring from the site this evening and it's more uncomfortable. Her mother told her to go and have it looked at right away, so here she is. She's got a small abscess where the earring was. I drain it and put her on an antibiotic.

This is followed by a 22-year-old white female with tooth pain. She had two teeth extracted earlier in the day. She has advanced periodontal disease, but I'm not finding much else. I need to get her out of here quickly so I put her on an antibiotic, and gave her a stronger pain med. She can follow up with her dentist.

Our 39-year-old with the belly pain for 30 minutes has completely normal lab and films. She is cured with Ativan (a tranquilizer). We'll treat symptomatically for now and have her follow-up as needed.

And the squad is out on yet another person with chest pain.

One of the Emergency Department nurses called the police to see what became of the juvenile they were bringing in. They're not coming in after all.

We've also got an 18-year-old white female with mid-back pain that began while she was driving. It's worse with movement and bending, but helped with Rolaids (why she tried Rolaids is beyond me). There's no history of trauma, and she's got reproducible mid-back paraspinous tenderness. I'll do a therapeutic X-ray, and give her my back potion (Toradol and Valium).

Meanwhile, the squad arrives. It's the chest pain we heard about. It's a 75-year-old white male who had a heart attack about 4 months ago that required emergent catheterization and angioplasty. This is the first chest pain he's had since the angioplasty, and it's just like his prior heart pain. He had three nitroglycerine at home, and a fourth in the squad. He arrives pain free. His EKG is nonspecific, and his lab is normal. Given the risk factors, he's admitted for a cardiac evaluation. This is unstable angina until proven otherwise, and could even be early reocclusion of his angioplastied vessels.

3:30 AM

And we've yet another person with chest pain coming in by squad. This is a person who was just recently discharged after some cardiac problems. I'm sure I'll get more information when they get here.

And of course our 18-year-old girl with back pain has normal films. She's feeling better with my concoction. I put her on back medicines and send her on her way.

And what did I say about the weather. I see a 45-year-old frequent flyer asthmatic in with exacerbation of her asthma. She's usually in because she leaves her medicines at home. She's also complaining of headache tonight, so her asthma can't be that bad. I call respiratory down to give her a treatment, and give her some routine headache medicines. She ultimately goes home happy.

The squad arrives, and the chest pain is a 66-year-old white male who was awakened with chest pain, shortness of breath, and bilateral arm radiation. He had a positive cardiac stress test a week ago, and a heart catheterization just a few days ago with diffuse disease. This guy is a keeper as well.

His EKG is nonspecific. I put him on routine cardiac medicines, and he's rapidly pain free.

Okay, our 29-year-old with the flank pain has a normal IVP. He became pain free in the Radiology suite. He likely passed a stone there. We'll send him home with some pain pills, a urine strainer (to catch the stone), and the recommendation to drink plenty of fluids. He can follow-up with either his local doctor or the urologist.

Our 66-year-old with chest pain is admitted early. He had an uneventful stay in the ER.

We then receive a 31-year-old white male with a 2 year history of "breathing problems." He's also had a sore shoulder for a couple of weeks. None of these symptoms are any worse, but he sees doctor NONE, and has decided that it is time to have them looked into. He tells me, "I wanted to wait until after the bar crowd," so he comes in at 0430 AM.

Oh lovely, a triple beeper. It's blue haired grandma with breathing problems. What did I say? This is an 81-year-old white female with a long history of asthma. Her breathing has been worse in the last couple of days. There seems to be a big component of anxiety. A breathing treatment, some steroids, a tranquilizer, and a therapeutic X-ray and we get her out of here.

6:00 AM

Zzzz...

Wow, almost three hours of sleep, but now I get to pay. The morning crowds are here in force. We have an 81-year-old white female who just had a CEA (a carotid endarterectomy, where the big artery in the neck is repaired or replaced) a couple of days ago and is complaining of shortness of breath.

In addition we have a 40-year-old white male who was "bit by a spider" three weeks ago and now has redness ascending his arm from the wound. Of course the type of bug in this case is a moot point. He's got a local cellulitis with lymphangitis. I put him on some Keflex (an antibiotic that works well for typical skin infections), and send him on his way. Why is it that every mosquito bite is a "spider bite?" Who can say?

Back to our 81-year-old with the shortness of breath. She has some post surgical swelling but otherwise not much noteworthy. She is helped with a breathing treatment. Her symptoms could be anxiety related or she could have a little bronchospasm (spasm of the big airways) from being intubated for the surgery. I put her on some Combivent (a breathing medicine) for a few days. If it is bronchospasm it will help. If it is anxiety, by virtue of placebo effect, it will also help. She wants to go home, so I sent her on her way.

The cafeteria isn't open on weekend mornings, so I have a vending machine breakfast. This is sometimes better than anything you can get from the cafeteria, which doesn't say much for the cafeteria.

Next is a 62 year old white female with Parkinson's Disease (a movement disorder with tremor, unstable gait, slow movement) who, by virtue of her disease, has frequent falls. She fell last night and is complaining of right ankle pain. Her films are fine so we'll treat it as a sprain. More importantly, we need to try and minimize her future fall risk. One of these days she's likely to do some serious damage.

This is followed by a 22-year-old post-partum white female with a constant headache since having an epidural (spinal anesthesia). This is worse when she is up, and frequently resolves when she's lying flat. It sounds like a post lumbar puncture headache. This can be produced by a chronic leak of spinal fluid after the initial spinal tap. A blood patch is used to seal the breach. For this procedure, some of the patient's own blood is withdrawn and injected around the site of the original puncture. The blood clots and (hopefully) seals the leak. I get anesthesia on the case.

Meanwhile I get an 82-year-old white female who comes in by squad. She had a ground level fall at home and was unable to get up. X-ray shows a left femoral neck fracture. This is one of the more common hip fractures that occur with ground level falls in the elderly. This requires a surgery to fix. The doctor on-call for her regular doctor and the orthopedic surgeon are contacted. She is likely to be taken to surgery later today.

Next we've got a 43-year-old white male with the worst case of poison ivy I've seen this summer. One might ask what part of his skin surface isn't involved. Some prednisone (a steroid) and Atarax (a antihistamine) should get him feeling better quicker.

Anesthesia wants to wait a while longer on our lady with the spinal headache. They think it will resolve without the blood patch. They treat her with caffeine and a pain medicine. Some folks respond to this. She can follow-up with them.

Then I've got a 37-year-old road warrior. He had a tooth break off and now has increasing pain and left upper facial swelling. From the look of his teeth, he hasn't seen a dentist, possibly ever. The tooth is broken off at the gumline. He's also got a facial cellulitis (a skin infection). We'll put him on an antibiotic and some pain pills, but he really needs to see a dentist. Half the time these folks get to feeling better with the meds, and don't follow-up. Then we see them again and again.

Next is a 78-year-old white female with increasing back spasms for the last few days. She has no history of trauma, but she does have a history of a metastatic (widely spread) GI cancer. Her films are okay and have no evidence of cancer in her spine. I give her my routine back spasm meds, and she's cured. We'll put her on an anti-inflammatory and an anti-spasmodic, and she should do fine. She can follow up with her regular doctor.

We've also got a 31-year-old white female who is 3 days post-partum from a c-section. She's been having fever and pain. She's got redness and foul smelling drainage from the incision site. She's also been feeling lightheaded. There's an obvious wound infection with a cellulitis (a skin infection) extending up her abdomen and down into her groin. We do some lab, including blood cultures.

We've also got a 46-year-old white male with cough, occasional bloody sputum, and chest pain for a week. The pain has been unchanged and constant despite a wide range of activity. His EKG is normal, as is his lab and X-ray. This is most consistent with bronchitis. We'll get him treated, and he can follow-up as needed.

12:00 PM

Boy they just keep on coming. The offices are closed now, and so it's only going to get worse. I see a 22-year-old white female with "migraine headache." She was in two days ago with similar complaints. She was exhibiting bizarre behavior at that time. She's more appropriate today, although she seems depressed.

She gets my routine headache pack, and is sent packing.

Then a 23-year-old white male comes in by squad. He's had a lot of physical activity in the last couple of days, and he developed sudden onset of low back spasm while gardening. Now this is just pathetic. How bad can a spontaneous back spasm be in a 23-year-old? He gets my routine back pain meds and is sent on his way.

Back to our 31-year-old post-partum lady with the obvious wound infection. It looks like she may be septic. I have her admitted. She'll get IV antibiotics and be evaluated by her gynecologist.

Then on to a 40-year-old white male who crushed his left index finger changing an oil filter. We get a film and it's normal. He's treated symptomatically.

Folks are coming in fast and furious. I'm having a hard time keeping up with recording the basics for this record.

We've got a 79-year-old white male who comes in complaining of shortness of breath. He has a little cough and congestion. He's a tiny little guy with a history of congestive heart failure, and he does note that he's had a three pound weight gain over the last day. He's had no chest pain or other significant signs or symptoms. Everything is unremarkable with the exception of some mild failure on the chest X-ray. The impression is that he's gotten a respiratory illness, a bronchitis, and his heart failure has decompensated slightly. This is something pretty frequently seen. It really doesn't require admission. The patient has a known history of failure, has had a non-cardiac event that can make it worse, and is not hypoxic. I bump up his Demodex (a diuretic or water pill) and put him on an antibiotic plus a cough medicine. I'll have him follow-up first of the week.

Another impression I get with this patient is that he is lonely, and wants someone to talk to. He lives alone. This is a frequent issue with the elderly. They often have outlived their friends and have no family nearby. They don't want to be in assisted living or a nursing home, but want to stay in their home. They get scared or lonely and come to the emergency room to socialize. They frequently create or exaggerate symptoms trying to get admitted. This way they get to have someone look after them for a few days. They are usually very resistant to nursing home stays, because they view that as where people go to die. I can't say that I blame them much.

The next patient I see is a 17-year-old white male with poison ivy. I think the last straw for this kid is that he's managed to get it all over his penis as well as his arms and legs. I put him on my usual steroid and anti-histamine combination. He should do fine. Boy I'm getting tired of this poison ivy stuff.

Then I have an 86-year-old white female with right shoulder pain. She's brought in by her daughter who appears to be the person in charge. Apparently there was a fall several weeks ago. They had seen their regular doctor but are not happy with what he had said or done. The daughter wants a "second opinion" and is insistent on an X-ray. There had been one done after the initial injury, but hey, we're here to please. Of course the film is fine. I wind up doing about 45 minutes of PR work. She's already on an anti-inflammatory medicine, and a mild pain medicine, but hasn't been taking them appropriately. I make arrangements for some physical therapy, which appeases the daughter. Another happy customer…

Then we've got a 3-year-old white female who ran into the edge of a dresser at home. She's got a small laceration on her face just lateral to her right eye. It's just big enough that it needs to be sutured. Talk about a challenge. Three is an age where it is just about impossible to reason with a child. You wind up having to strap them down on a papoose board and just press on. The only part that hurts at all is the initial numbing, but they usually scream from that point on. This child is no exception. She gets her stitches and is sent on her way.

You really have to wonder about folks' perception of the term "emergency." Next is a 36-year-old white male with bilateral foot pain. He's a factory worker and spends a lot of time on his feet. For the last several weeks the soles of his feet hurt at the end of the day. When he went on a vacation the pain went away. He's back on the job, and his feet hurt again. This is not rocket science, and this is not a Saturday afternoon emergency. He needs some better shoes and maybe an anti-inflammatory for a while.

Then we have a 39-year-old white male who was disassembling a truck rack at home when a piece fell on him and cut his scalp. You would swear this guy was like the 3-year-old with the facial laceration. He was just spazzing out about getting sutured. This was little more than a scratch, and really didn't need anything.

This was followed by a 16-year-old white male with 3 day history of fever, sore throat and frontal headache. His exam was normal and his strep screen was negative. This is a viral sore throat. He could have mononucleosis. I've seen a lot of it. However, mono is just treated symptomatically as well. Unless they insist, or are real dramatic, I don't always test for it. He just needs to treat this symptomatically for a while. I try to steer folks like this away from antibiotics. Sometimes I'm successful, sometimes not. It all depends on their agenda and their perception of what is appropriate medical care.

Then I'm back to another 3-year-old with a right eyebrow laceration. Same song different verse; same chapter different page. We get it sutured among the cries and wails.

I love my job, I love my job…

The end is in sight. My shift is nearing a close, but not before a few more people wander in…

We have a 10-month-old with three days of a fever and nasal drainage. The exam is normal. I get the impression that these are first-time parents. They are just sure that something bad is going on. The kid, for the most part, is smiling and happy. I order some lab so it seems like I'm doing something. Appearances are everything. I can't count the number of therapeutic labs and X-rays I do. We'll see.

Meanwhile I get a 23-year-old white male who rolled his 4 wheeler. Of course he was wearing no protective gear. At least he was going very slowly when it happened, but he did take the weight of the bike across his pelvis. He walked in under his own power, but was looking pretty stiff and sore. I ordered a range of tests.

While waiting, I see a 14 year old who cut his right long finger on a can. It's relatively superficial, but does gape when he flexes his finger. He's never had a stitch before and thinks it is really cool how he has no sensation once the finger is numbed. I put in a few stitches and send him on his way.

My relief shows up a bit early. This is about the time our rollover victim's films come back. He's got a stable pelvic fracture on the left, but my relief thinks he sees something on the right. He wants to go ahead and take over the patients in progress, which is fine with me.

I get back to my tall stack of dictation. I work at this for the next 45 minutes or so. Peripherally I hear that the 10-month-old child's lab just looks viral, surprise! The rollover victim, after another thousand dollars worth of CT scanning and the like, has no other injuries. They both go home, and so did I…

6:00 PM

Shift 12
"They're sucking the life out of me!"

Sunday—18 Hours

12:00 PM

What a zoo. The rooms are all full. Four admits are stacked up, and more folks keep pouring in. My first thought is that I'd like to just turn around and get out of here. No such luck...

I'm taking over a 28-year-old white male who I saw a few days ago. I diagnosed pneumonia, and given his indigent status I arranged for a full course of antibiotic. He is back and doesn't feel he's been getting better. He's had a complete reevaluation and doesn't have any specific criteria for admission so far.

Well, the final test came back on our pneumonia guy, and is normal. The prior shift was not yet out the door and they finished him up, and arranged follow-up.

Then I've got a 16-year-old white male who mashed his finger in the car door last night. He's got a subungual hematoma (a collection of blood under the nail), but no fracture. I drained the hematoma with cautery, and this should make him feel better.

Second, I've also got a 31-year-old white female who has a history of multiple ectopic pregnancies (a fetus in a place it doesn't belong, like in the fallopian tubes) in the past. She's having mid-cycle spotting that she says is exactly how her ectopics have presented in the past.

Third, there's a 78-year-old white female who just doesn't feel well. She's had some nausea for a week. She's also had a chronic urinary infection. We'll check it out and see what we find. I give her some Compazine (an anti-nausea medicine) to try and get her feeling better while we wait.

Fourth, there's a 63 year old white female with poison ivy on her face. She's got quite a lot of poison ivy in her yard and didn't initially realize it. I put her on some prednisone (a steroid) and Atarax (an antihistamine). She can follow-up as needed.

Fifth, there's an 89 year old white female with an infected leg for the last two weeks. She was brought in because there were maggots crawling on her. She's got open sores on her left leg with maggots in the wound. She is filthy. It makes me wonder if she ever gets a bath or shower. She's obviously demented. I really wonder about safety at home given her current condition.

From this point on this shift, I'm recording retrospectively. The whole shift went to hell in a hand-basket. I pretty much worked continuously 18 hours non-stop. When I finally got home, I collapsed for about three hours, and now that I am feeling at least semi-human, I'll try and capture the essence of what happened. I was able to at least jot down the sequence in which I saw things, but time became a blur. All right…

Our 89-year-old has a cellulitis of her left leg with ulcers that are being cleaned by the maggots. If the home situation was not so suspect, this type of infection could be treated with outpatient antibiotics. The local doctor wants us to have her placed in a nursing home. We spent forever trying to arrange this, but it's almost impossible to accomplish on a Sunday. We finally talk him in to admitting her overnight. She can go to the nursing home tomorrow.

There's an 18-year-old white female with a sore throat for several days. We'll see what the strep test shows.

Meanwhile we have a 22-year-old white male who twisted his ankle coming down a stairway. He complains of left lateral foot pain. His films are fine. He should respond to routine treatment.

Our 31-year-old who was worried about ectopic pregnancy is not pregnant, and so it's pretty hard for her to have an ectopic pregnancy. She is skeptical of our ultra sensitive pregnancy test, but there's not much I can do about that. She does have microscopic hematuria (blood in the urine), and is already on Bactrim (an antibiotic). She just needs to follow-up in a week or two to make sure the urine has cleared.

Our 18-year-old with the sore throat has a negative strep. She's got a viral sore throat. This is symptomatic treatment unless they just demand an antibiotic. She seems appeased with the testing we've done.

Next is a 40-year-old white male who's gotten food stuck in his throat. He isn't tolerating his own secretions. He tells us this has happened before. When it does, he's needed endoscopic removal. It doesn't help my nurses' peace of mind that he's got about every blood-born disease known to man. I decide to try medical management first. Frequently, if you can get the esophagus muscles to relax, it will pass on through. He gets some Ativan (a tranquilizer) and some Glucagon (a diabetes medicine that relaxes esophageal muscles as a side effect). Then we wait...

I've also got a 72-year-old white male who for the last half-hour has complete amnesia of the period covering the entire morning. He's done a range of things through the morning that he has absolutely no recollection of doing. Of course, he's looking a bit bewildered. He has no other focal findings. His wife related that this had happened once before, but that it had only lasted a few minutes. He's never had it looked into. The biggest concern is that this patient is having some type of brain event. I start our standard stroke work-up...

Meanwhile we have a tearful 18-year-old white female with a three day history of right-sided back pain. It's much worse today. Some lab had already been done and she has blood in her urine. An IVP is ordered. It'll take an hour to complete, so meanwhile I give her some IV fluids and some IV Toradol.

Then I see a 16 year old white male with an alleged "migraine headache." He really seems pretty darned comfortable. His exam is normal. I give him some routine headache medicines, and then the real agenda comes out. He wants a note to get off work. Fine, whatever. What an expensive way to get a note for work.

Hmmm. We'll see if things run in threes today. I have a 19-year-old tearful white female with sudden onset right flank pain and blood in her urine. Her family is wigging out as much as she is, and so I have to spend time calming everyone down. They really project this sense of entitlement. The emergency room is completely overflowing, and they seem to think that they should be taken care of first. Whatever…This girl is having some vomiting as well. I get her some IV fluids, Toradol, and Compazine. We're backed up in X-ray so she has to wait. The Toradol isn't adequate, so she gets some Demerol. She's in the queue for an IVP (a contrast dye exam of her kidney and its collecting system). Her regular doctor shows up even though he's not on call. My impression is that the family called him from the lobby because they felt things weren't going quickly enough for their satisfaction. Surprisingly, he backed me up, provided some reassurance to the family, and left us to do what we do.

Meanwhile there's a 42-year-old white female with one day of low back pain. It's worse with bending and moving. There's no history of trauma, no radiation, no weakness or numbness. Her exam is normal except for some muscle tenderness in back. Here also, the family is acting like she's dying. I order some therapeutic lab and X-rays, and give her my usual back sprain concoction, Toradol and Valium. Then we wait…

Next door is a 39-year-old white male with abdominal pain for a day. It started around his belly button and has migrated to his right lower abdomen. He's nauseated, and has a low-grade fever. He's got exquisite point tenderness in his right lower abdomen. This is appendicitis until proven otherwise. The doctor on-call for this patient just happens to be in the emergency room admitting another patient, and he concurs. The surgeon is called in and he is off to surgery.

Then I zip over to see a 6-year-old white male who had a roller blading accident. He fell and wound up with some road rash on his right knee and the back of his right hand. Of course he was wearing no protective gear, it just "isn't cool." Well, he's paying for it now. There's nothing to sew. He's cleaned up and sent on his way.

We've also got a 39-year-old white male who races motorcycles. He fell off one earlier in the day and has right rib and hip pain. The hip is fine, but he has a nasty set of rib fractures. Luckily, he hasn't collapsed a lung, but given the appearance of the fractures, it is still a possibility. The surgeon is in seeing the appendicitis, so I had him give me his impression. He concurred that this just needs follow-up. I put him on some pain meds and he can see his regular doctor.

Meanwhile we get the rest of the results back from our 72-year-old with amnesia. We're not really finding anything. He is able to remember things told him since his arrival, but the morning is lost. His regular doctor wants to send him out on Aspirin and Plavix (mild blood thinners), but I'm a little uncomfortable with this. This is at least a TIA and possibly a stroke. I've never seen one present quite like this. We compromise on getting the neurologists opinion. The neurologist feels this was a TIA involving posterior circulation of the brain, and since the patient is able to retain short-term memory now and has no other deficits, that Aspirin, Plavix, and outpatient management is appropriate. The patient and his wife are completely okay with this. We get him the first dose of meds, and let him leave with follow-up.

I swing by a 13-year-old who injured his left wrist hooking up a boat to a trailer. He's got a buckle fracture of his radius and ulna (the main bones of his forearm). This is just a little twist in the bone rather than a through and through fracture. It's splinted and they can been seen in follow-up.

Back to our 18-year-old girl with the right-sided back pain. She was completely pain free. She had had a distal partial obstruction on the IVP initially, that cleared during the study. She has likely passed a stone. She can strain her urine and be seen as an outpatient.

Our 19-year-old with the left flank pain also passed a stone during the IVP and is pain free. She too can strain her urine and be seen as an outpatient.

The 40-year-old with the food stuck in his throat gets another dose of glucagon (this is a hyperglycemic agent that also incidentally relaxes the esophagus) with no improvement. The surgeon is called out to scope him. Just before the surgeon gets in to see the patient, the food goes on down and the patient is cured. Another save! He needs to eat smaller bites. He also needs further evaluation to see why he continues to have this problem.

I doubt he will follow-up.

Our 42-year-old with the back pain has normal lab and films of course. She still is complaining of a lot of pain. I give her some Nubain (a non-narcotic pain medicine) which has her floating and feeling no pain. I start her on my routine back pain regimen. In this case it's Daypro, Flexeril, and Vicodin (an anti-inflammatory, a muscle relaxant, and pain medicine). She can follow-up as needed.

Okay, at least I'm freeing up some rooms. Time to get back into the fray…

We've got a 23-year-old white female who fell off her bike while jumping her bike off a ramp. She complains of right hip pain. Her films are normal. She's just bruised her hip as well as her ego.

Hmmm. We've got this three thing creeping up again. Next is a 58-year-old white female who has a history of TIA and presents with several hours of left-sided numbness and left arm weakness. She's already on aspirin and Plavix (platelet active blood thinners). Her work-up is unremarkable except for an elevated sedimentation rate. This test is a marker of inflammation that can be elevated in such things as vasculitis (inflammation of blood vessels), a disorder than can cause stroke like symptoms. At the very least she is having a TIA, at the worst, a stroke or vasculitis. She warrants admission, and we get her going.

Bingo. Here's the third, a 77-year-old white female with sudden onset of the inability to find words. The symptoms have been present for several hours, and are slowly improving. She's had a similar episode several months previously that lasted only a few minutes. It was investigated without specific findings. She was on no stroke preventatives except her blood pressure medicines. Her work-up here is negative, and her symptoms completely cleared. We get her an aspirin and a Plavix (both act as platelet inhibitors and reduce stroke risk). We paged her regular doctor to coordinate follow-up, and then encountered a monkey wrench in the system. Her symptoms returned. In addition, she now has left facial drooping. Hold the presses. She gets admitted.

And we're back to the mundane. Next is a 25-year-old white male with a migraine headache. He's taken nothing for it of course. He gets my cocktail, and again the agenda comes out. He wants off work for the day. I give him what he wants.

Then we have a 3-year-old white male who fell backward after sliding down a slide and caught his scalp on a sharp edge. He has a tiny superficial laceration, but the mother insists that it keeps bleeding. It's not bleeding. I wind up putting a single skin staple in it just to appease the mother.

Next is a 32-year-old white female who ran a 26-mile marathon in the heat and humidity. Following this, she's weak and lightheaded. Her electrolytes are fine. A liter of IV fluid and she's ready to go. Looks like some simple heat exhaustion.

A problem that I was facing solved itself. Several days ago I had seen a 20-year-old white male and his pregnant girlfriend. He was having burning with urination. His urinalysis was negative, but I talked him into a test for gonorrhea and chlamydia. He refused empiric treatment and wanted to wait for the results. There was no way to get in touch with him or his girlfriend directly, and of course his test came back positive for chlamydia. Well he called earlier in the day for results, and then showed up for treatment. Of course he still sees doctor NONE, and has made no effort to obtain a local doctor. We give him his meds so we know he is treated, and send him on his way.

His 21-year-old pregnant girlfriend also showed up. She wants to be treated as well and gets the same treatment. She is also complaining of left ear pain and is put on cortisporin (a combination ear medicine). She had had a urinary infection when seen previously, and had not gotten her prescription filled or followed-up as recommended. Recall that she had the stent for kidney stone that still needs to be removed in addition to the newly verified pregnancy. We rechecked her and she is still infected. We give her some antibiotic samples, and a script for a cheaper antibiotic. Her boyfriend said he would fill it. We also made arrangements for social services to get involved. She has no job, no resources, is apparently breaking up with her dirt-bag boyfriend, and is pregnant. Lovely combination, and surely soon to be on our Welfare roles. Ah well, you can't win them all.

On to something real, a 52-year-old white male who tripped and fell down some stairs. He's got left hip and thigh pain and is unable to bear weight. He's fractured his hip. Fortuitously, the orthopedic surgeon called at this time. He was about to go out of town for a few hours and wanted to see if there was any business. Yes...

Then we had a tragedy. A 22-year-old white male who drowned while swimming in one of the local swimming mud holes. He was under the water for well over an hour and a half. There was really nothing to be done except to pronounce him dead.

Next is a 67-year-old white male with a ten day history of rash on his left arm. He's convinced himself he has Lyme disease, and if he doesn't get it looked after right away he will surely die or worse. He's got a little dermatitis. I offer a Lyme titer, but once I explain his near zero relative risk, he feels reassured and wants to follow-up with his regular doctor.

Then we have a 54-year-old white male who was pinched between the family boat and the dock when a cable came loose. He is having some back pain. His films were fine so I treated him for contusion and send him on his way.

6:00 PM

This was followed by a 69-year-old white female who had a ground level fall this morning and is having left knee pain. She came in by squad and wants to be admitted. She feels she just can't get along at home. Her films showed arthritis. I tell her that all we could really justify would be a nursing home until she is on her feet. She was agreeable to this. She still winds up getting admitted for the night with follow-up placement in the morning.

To contrast this is a 73-year-old white female who fell backwards and is having left groin pain. She had a history of both hips being replaced and she walks haltingly with a walker. She can't support herself with her arms alone. Her films show a new stable pelvic fracture, but she wants to go home. We try to get her adequately pain controlled so she could walk and get along at home, but are unable. She'll need placement for a few weeks.

What a rush, and the fun just doesn't stop...

Well, the family of the drowning victim came in and I had to break the news that their loved one was indeed dead. This was followed by a lot of screaming and throwing things around the room. Thankfully we were able to get everyone calmed down, on their way, and the body to the mortuary in about three hours.

We then got a call of an 87-year-old white female coming over from one of the nursing homes with abdominal pain due to constipation. Well, this woman looked on death's doorstep. She was ashen, marginally responsive, hypoxic, and had a belly that looked like a beach ball. There were no bowel sounds present. She was not impacted, or overly constipated. I verified quickly just how aggressive we were going to have to be by talking with the family. Thankfully they wanted no aggressive measures. Once I saw her chest X-ray, I knew we were in trouble. She had huge air under her diaphragm. She had probably infarcted her bowel and had it perforate. Then the lab came back and was looking incompatible with life, and I quickly painted the picture for the family of just how grim things looked. I called the regular doctor, and he arrived just as the patient expired.

We also have a 48-year-old white male with chest and upper abdominal pressure. He's hypertensive and a diabetic. His symptoms have been going on intermittently through the weekend. It's worse with any exertion and better with rest. He has an episode in the Emergency Department that is cured by nitroglycerine. All the cardiac work-up was unremarkable. He is given cardiac protective meds despite this. Given his risk factors, this patient has cardiac disease until proven otherwise. He wanted his regular doctor from a nearby city to manage his case. His regular doctor refused transfer, giving a lame excuse. Reading between the lines, the impression was that he was busy, and didn't want any more work this evening. He indicated he would be more than happy to provide follow-up after the patient was fully evaluated by our cardiologists. Nice guy. Just the sort you want to look after you.

9:00 PM

Well there's got to be a three-fer here with the next few cases. They're car wrecks. We've got a 12-year-old white male who was a restrained passenger in a car that was rear-ended at a stoplight. He complains of some neck stiffness and some left groin pain. His exam is unremarkable. We do films that are fine. He has sprains and bruises. He'll do fine.

The mother is a 32-year-old white female who was a restrained passenger in the front. She is complaining of neck stiffness, left knee pain, and low back pain. She also has bumps and bruises. They are both advised and discharged.

Then we've got a sad case, a 58-year-old black female with widely metastatic cancer of the pancreas. She's been on pretty big-gun narcotics for pain and is constipated to beat the band. She gets multiple enemas before it starts to break loose. We give her something to drink at home to finish the job. This person has no future; it's sad.

Then we see an 18-year-old white female with a typical Welfare attitude. She's had some diffuse abdominal pain for a week and chooses midnight to have it looked into. She works at UNEM and sees doctor NONE. When asked why she hadn't seen someone earlier in the week, she said in no uncertain terms that she had Medicaid, and that it allowed her to see whomever she wanted whenever she wanted. What a waste of taxpayer money. So, in the end, she's constipated. What could have been solved for $5 at the local grocery store, winds up costing $500 at the local Emergency Room. Go figure...

Then we have a 4-year-old white female with a sore throat for 45 minutes. I want to pull my hair out. This kids exam is normal, the strep screen is negative, she doesn't even complain of a sore throat. Get out of here...

Well I'm sure this must be the third car wreck. It's a 34-year-old white female who was a restrained driver in a MVA. She has neck pain. Films are fine, so I put her on my usual sprain medicines and send her on her way.

The next case is weird. It's a 47-year-old white female brought in by squad. She's drunk, she fell about one foot from her deck, and has no complaints. So why is she here? And by squad at that? Who knows? After a quick exam, I get her out the door.

Well it looks like yet another three-fer. It's a 17-year-old white female with low back pain and difficulty urinating. She's got blood in her urine and gets the same course as the two before her. IVP shows distal partial obstruction. She winds up pain free, and gets to go home to pee through a strainer.

12:00 AM

Then we've got a 13-year-old white female who feels "shaky." She's also complaining of sharp chest pain with a deep breath. She was out all evening with "friends." She looks like she's taken some methamphetamine (speed, crank), but she denies this. I am dubious. I do a full evaluation, including drug screen, and it's all unremarkable. I'm surprised. I get so used to people lying to me it's almost amazing when they're actually tell the truth. I give her a Xanax (a tranquilizer) and she's cured. Perhaps this was some type of anxiety reaction. I'll let her follow up with her regular doctor.

Then we have another non-emergency, a 19-year-old white female who was diagnosed with mononucleosis about a week ago. She's miserable. She hurts all over. She's got a world class sore throat. She can't sleep. In the end, I get her some symptomatic medicines so she can sleep.

For the first time since I came on shift, I've actually cleared out the ER. I've had no opportunity to do any of the paperwork, so now I'm dictating to beat the band.

One of the local police stopped by off duty. His wife is very pregnant, and she got mad when he wasn't ready to go to sleep and wanted to watch TV. He stopped by to escape for a while.

3:00 AM

Shit, shit, shit. The dictation system went down. Ah well, patients are starting to roll in again anyway.

We've got a 69-year-old white male who had sudden onset lower abdominal pain starting at midnight. This is followed by repeated vomiting and diarrhea. Then he began to pass out every time he vomited or sat upright. Initially it seemed like a simple of case of a stomach bug, some dehydration, and a strong vagus response. I gave him some fluids, and some nausea medicine. Even with this though, every time we sat him up he passed out and vomited. Then his blood pressure began to drift down despite the fluids. Lab was relatively unremarkable. Cardiac evaluation was unremarkable. He didn't appear to be bleeding into his bowel. He was getting a lot of fluid, and we continued to make no progress in either figuring out what was going on or improving his status.

Something I learned in residency, when you haven't got a clue what's going on and the patient is crashing, it's time to spread the wealth. I called the patient's doctor and got him and his resident on the case. After 18 hours my diagnostic acumen well is dry. I let them take over.

Oh, one final annoyance. In the middle of all this the 21-year-old white female that I had treated for chlamydia exposure came back. She had been seen by one of my partners the night before with her ear infection. He'd actually given her a shot of Demerol for this. She came back at exactly the same time, to the minute, expecting to see him again. I think she was expecting another shot of Demerol. Not...He had also given her a script for some Vicodin (a mild narcotic) that she did not fill. I give her a four pack of Vicodin and tell her to hit the road. I know she is going to keep coming back. She's going to become the bane of our existence.

I love my job. I love my job.

6:00 AM

I stayed a half-hour over to finish my dictation using my partner's account, then I was gone.

Shift 13
"Veterinary Medicine..."

Tuesday—18 Hours

6:00 PM

It sounds like the previous shift was a zoo. Hopefully the trend doesn't continue. There's nothing that was passed off, so I start with a clean slate. However, it doesn't last for long.

Clinic starts with a 10-year-old white male who had his left thumb stepped on while playing football. His film is fine. He needs to be treated symptomatically.

Next is a 27-year-old white male who was literally screwing around last weekend. He was having unprotected sex. Now he's got some pain with urination and is worried about the clap. Of course he works at UNEM and sees doctor NONE. I do the swab, and convince him to be treated empirically. He can follow-up later, though it is doubtful that he will.

Then we've got a 66 year old white male who had a heart catheterization about a week ago. He's now got an increasing swelling in his right groin. He's also on Coumadin (a blood thinner). Two things we need to check. First, what is his protime (the measure of blood thinness). Second is to ensure there is no pseudoaneurysm.

When people have a heart catheterizations, a plastic catheter is placed in the femoral artery in their groin. When the procedure is finished, the catheter is removed, and pressure is applied to ensure the wound clots shut. Sometimes the man-made defect in the artery doesn't seal over properly and the high pressure arterial blood makes its own track into the leg. When this occurs it is referred to as a pseudoaneurysm, and it sometimes requires surgical repair. I send him off for ultrasound to see if this complication has occurred.

In the meantime I've got a 17-year-old white male that injured his left forearm playing football. He's convinced it's broken because he heard a "pop." There's no deformity and only minimal tenderness. Of course the films are fine. He's bruised his arm.

Back to our groin swelling. The ultrasound took just a few minutes and is fine. There's a hematoma, a collection of blood under the skin, but no pseudoaneurysm. This is no big deal. His protime is not quite even therapeutic. This just needs to be treated symptomatically. The hematoma will resorb, but not before he has one hummer of a bruise.

Then we've got one of our regulars. It's, surprise, a 27-year-old white female complaining of migraine headache. We've been seeing her much more frequently lately. It always seems to be in the evening, a couple of hours after the doctor's offices are closed. Of course she's got a nice list of "allergies." I give her my usual, and kick her out the door.

Next is a 72-year-old white female here with her suitcase (this is known as the positive suitcase sign). She was seen in the office today because she "just doesn't feel well." She had a chest X-ray and EKG there because of some vague chest discomfort. She was put on an antibiotic and some steroids for a presumed bronchitis. She's complaining of "chest tightness." She wants to be admitted, and has managed to hit on the right words to say in order to accomplish her mission. Actually I'm rather surprised that more people don't figure this out. Of course everything we check is normal, she's likely got a virus, but she's admitted regardless.

Boy we just go from one crisis to another. Next is a 22-year-old white male with a four day history of poison ivy on his legs. It's an emergency now. I guess he figures it's going to make it hard to sleep tonight. I give him my usual, steroids and antihistamines, and send him packing.

Then there's a 10-day-old white female with low grade fever. She's got an apparent left otitis media (ear infection). Given the age we do other lab to ensure nothing else is going on. Her current temperature is 99^3 rectal. The magic number for a sepsis work-up is 100^5. I've mentioned this before. Babies one month and under have a significant risk of serious infection, much higher than older children, when they run fevers.

What a spectrum, pediatrics to geriatrics. Next is a 84-year-old white female who tripped on the sidewalk and fell. She bumped her head and sustained a laceration across the bridge of her nose. There was no loss of consciousness, and she has no other specific complaint except for her nose. It looks pretty uncomfortable. The X-ray shows that she did manage to break it pretty good. I stitch her up. She'll have to see the Ear, Nose and Throat folks tomorrow.

Then we have a 36-year-old black female who's had insulin dependent diabetes for 10 years. She stopped taking her insulin a month ago because she'd been having low blood sugars. She hasn't talked to her regular doctor about this, and she hasn't been checking her blood sugars. Now she's been nauseated and light headed for the last couple of days. Her blood sugar is out of sight. No surprise there. The remainder of her lab, including serum ketones, are negative, and so she's not in diabetic ketoacidosis. We give her some IV fluids and some insulin and get both resolution of her symptoms and significant improvement of her blood sugar. She will follow-up with her doctor in the morning to get restarted on treatment of her diabetes.

We've also got a 20-year-old white female with angioedema. She's had sudden onset facial swelling while outside. She's had no specific exposures that she is aware of, and has never had this happen before. She's pretty puffy, but is having no breathing difficulties. We get her some Decadron, some Vistaril, and a breathing treatment. Then we watch her for a while…

We've also got a 79-year-old obese white female with sudden onset chest and left arm pain. Her pain occurred at rest, and she has not taken a nitroglycerine pill. She has known coronary artery disease, and has just had multiple heart vessels angioplastied and stented. She is cured with single sublingual nitroglycerine in our department. The EKG shows new onset atrial fibrillation and she does have elevated heart enzymes. She's a keeper. She's probably having a little heart attack. Her doctor is notified, and she's quickly admitted.

It's almost midnight, so of course we get a 21-year-old white male with mid-chest sharp pain. He's sure he's having a heart attack. The pain's reproducible with pushing on his chest. He had just started weight lifting today so he could "get in shape" for a new job, and he essentially pulled some muscles in his chest. He then spazzed out. He's cured with Toradol and Xanax, an anti-inflammatory and a tranquilizer. What a nut. Working at this job, it seems that people completely lose their ability to use common sense. Isn't it more likely that the chest pain and tenderness you have after a vigorous workout might be just because you overdid it? Prior to leaving this guys biggest concern is that he get a work release so he can stay home from work tonight.

The final patient before the witching hour is a 20-year-old with right ear pain for 3 or 4 days. He's got an otitis media (ear infection) and otitis externa (ear canal infection). He gets Amoxicillin (an antibiotic), Cortisporin (a combination ear drop) and some Tylenol with codeine.

12:00 AM

Midnight, and the deck has been cleared.
Zzzz…

2:15 AM

Crisis time, it's a 74-year-old white male with sudden onset of an itchy rash on his wrists. It's pretty much gone by the time I see him. Then his real issue comes out. He's had a recent small stroke, and he's been having intermittent headaches. He was worried that this means he was having more strokes. I provide some reassurance and send him on his way.

Zzzz…

5:00 AM

The 19-year-old white female I'd seen this weekend with right flank pain is back. She'd had a kidney stone that she passed during an IVP. She went home with follow-up. The next day she had another episode of flank pain and passed a second stone. Well she's got the same symptoms now. She's got large blood in the urine, so this becomes something of a no brainer. It takes quite a bit of narcotic to keep her comfortable. I chat with her regular doctor and she's admitted.

This is followed, almost immediately, by a 25-year-old white male with sudden onset right flank pain. It looks like we're trying to shoot for another three-fer. His pain's better with Toradol and Compazine. He too has large blood in his urine. We'll get an IVP and see what it shows.

Boy clinic is starting early this morning. We've got a 28-year-old white male with a "migraine headache." He's another frequent visitor to our department, though we haven't seen him for several months. He's better with Toradol, Phenergan, and DHE, so he's out of here. Of course, the last thing he asks for before going out the door is a work release. It does make you wonder, doesn't it?

Like I've said before, we should just leave blank signed forms in the lobby. Then half these folks probably wouldn't check in.

Boy, everyone is waking up. The next patient is a little 98-year-old grandma from the nursing home. She has some neck pain this morning and didn't want to get out of bed. Because of this the nursing home sent her in to be sure she didn't have a stroke. Go figure. I sure don't see the association there. On exam, I'm not really seeing anything except for some right sided neck tenderness. She's demented to beat the band, and she's confused and upset about being away from her home. We're pretty much obligated to scan her because of the Nursing Home concerns, but then we should be able to send her back. You know, even if we found something, what are we going to do? Why nothing of course.

More Nursing Home madness follows. Next is a 79-year-old white female sent over from the Nursing Home with low back pain and an elevated blood sugar. She's had low back pain off and on for years, and this is no different. Also, she's a diabetic and hasn't had her insulin yet. One would expect her blood sugar to be elevated. Ah well, we're still obligated to investigate this stuff. We need to make sure she hasn't got a urinary tract infection, a spontaneous compression fracture, or the like.

Our 98-year-old can go back to the nursing home. Her scan was fine, as is her lab. She may have had a TIA, but it's not evident at this time. We'll put her on an aspirin a day, and have her follow-up. As I indicated, it doesn't make sense to do a complete stroke work-up in a demented 98-year-old. If we were to find, for example, that she has narrowed carotid arteries, no surgeon would take her in to do a carotid endarterectomy and clean those arteries out. I send her back.

Next we've got a common injury, a 6-year-old white male whose left long finger was caught in the bathroom door during a squabble with his sister over bathroom rights. It's amputated the distal tip of his finger. We'll see what the films look like. I'll probably need the orthopedic surgeon to take a look.

Oh Joy, the return of our 28-year-old white non-compliant indigent diabetic with the pneumonia. He was here the day before yesterday. He was also at a regional medical center yesterday, as well as about a week ago. He says he can't breath. He wants to be admitted. Again he sees doctor NONE and works at UNEM. Given the number of ER visits, I'm pretty much obligated to pull out the stops to verify that nothing else is going on. He's had multiple labs, multiple X-rays, and a lower leg ultrasound over the past week. Except for X-ray findings, everything has been negative so far.

Our 6-year-old is going to be taken to surgery to clean up the wound. He didn't fracture the bone in the finger, but he did expose the tip of it. He's just too worked up to take care of in the Emergency Department. Regardless, he's out of my ER. Boy, his sister is going to have a lot of making up to do.

We don't find much on our 79-year-old from the nursing home. She gets her insulin and goes back to the nursing home.

Our 28-year-old is becoming a diagnostic dilemma. He's had multiple oral and IV antibiotics and has progressive findings on the chest X-ray. He's borderline hypoxic and is hyperventilating. He has increasing effusions (fluid under the lungs), increasing consolidation, and findings suggestive of heart failure. This guy has something serious going on that I'm not identifying. He's a keeper, if only because of all the ER visits. I outline the last several weeks course for the doctor who has taken care of him in the past, and he gets admitted to evaluate this further.

Changeover is coming soon, but first I've got an 84-year-old white male with a stroke history who comes in with new onset left sided weakness. This has been going on for the last several hours. He's already on aspirin and Aggranox (a platelet active blood thinner), and thus could be considered a failure on these medicines. The primary doctor had called ahead and just wanted us to look at him and report our findings. I do, and report back, and he was admitted directly.

There has to be at least one person who comes in just as my shift was ending. In this case it's a 73-year-old white female who was visiting a family member who had been admitted into another part of the hospital. She had passed out in the room and is now confused to beat the band. I start a stroke work-up on her, and check her out to the next shift.

12:00 PM

Enough for one shift, but not too bad overall. I am out of here...

Shift 14
"Boredom is a good thing!"

Friday—18 Hours

6:00 AM

I'm back...A little 90-year-old gentleman is passed off to me. He had experienced weakness, chest pressure, and shortness of breath starting at 4:00 AM. He's never had these symptoms before, which is surprising given his history. He was just in a couple weeks ago with new onset Atrial Fibrillation and Congestive Heart Failure. He's also had a recent positive stress test (a non-invasive test, like an exercise treadmill test, that uncovers coronary artery disease), and so has known ischemic heart disease. He is symptom free after a single nitroglycerine in the squad. His EKG shows new anterior/septal changes that suggests lack of adequate oxygen to that part of his heart. He's definitely a keeper. I've give some protective medicines and leave a message for his regular doctor to swing by when she shows up to make her morning rounds on the hospital floor.

Clinic begins and I see a 38-year-old white female with two weeks of cough, congestion, and increasing shortness of breath. Of course she's still smoking a pack and a half a day, and doesn't see any association between that and her lack of response to her current medical treatment. She had seen her doctor two days ago and was started on Levaquin (a good broad-spectrum antibiotic) and an inhaler. Of course she hasn't talked further with her regular doctor, and can't wait another hour to be seen in the office.

She's got diminished breath sounds, a harsh cough, and borderline oxygen saturation. I given her some steroids, a couple of breathing treatments, and get her queued up for a chest X-ray.

The 90-year-old has been stable. His lab and X-ray look fine. We've given him routine protective medicines, and he remains symptom free. His regular doctor stops by and admits him.

We've also got a 14-year-old white female who twisted her right ankle playing volleyball this morning. Once again, it couldn't wait until the doctor's office opens in 15 minutes. Her X-rays were normal, and he gets routine sprain instructions.

Our 38-year-old, meanwhile, has a normal chest X-ray. She's had dramatic improvement with a couple of nebulizer treatments. She was put on a prednisone (a steroid) taper, and started on nebulizer treatments through the week. It is reinforced that she needs to cut back on the smoking, but I'm sure that this fell on deaf ears. She's likely got spasm of her airways due to a combination of a viral respiratory illness and her smoking. This is likely why the antibiotic provided little improvement.

Then I see a 31-year-old white female who tripped in the yard last night and has multiple abrasions on both lower legs and her left knee. Her neighbor felt that the knee might require suturing. This is problematic as her wounds are really deep abrasions rather than lacerations. Given the fact that the injury occurred over 12 hours ago, risk of infection is increased, even if there was something to sew (The longer a wound remains open to the environment, the more likely it is to become contaminated with skin surface bacteria. If enough bacteria is in the wound and it is closed, you are essentially creating an abscess. This is NOT a good thing, obviously). She just needs routine wound care and instructions. Her tetanus is up to date. We clean her up, dress her wounds, and send her on the way.

11:00 AM

Hmmm. Kind of a lull here. As far as I'm concerned it can go on all day. As I frequently tell the nurses, "boredom is a good thing." Among other things, it means a lower likelihood of generating any significant litigation.

12:00 PM

And, all good things have to come to an end. I just got the word that someone is being wheeled in with back pain. Ah well…

Okay. We've got a 71-year-old white female, who has had some urinary discomfort for the last couple of days, and now comes in with 20 minutes of sharp left flank pain. She does have a distant history of kidney stones. Then, prior to giving a pain medicine, she has almost complete spontaneous resolution of her symptoms.

And then all hell breaks loose…

First we have a 53-year-old white male who ran a skill saw across his knee. He missed both the bone and major tendons in the area. It goes back together with 18 sutures.

Second for a two-fer we had a 62-year-old white male who fell into a glass case and shredded his right forearm. He didn't do any real serious damage, but it sure created a jigsaw puzzle to repair. 25 sutures later and he is back together.

Third we have a 2-year-old white female who swallowed an unknown number of Orudis (ketoprofen, an arthritis medicine). Apparently her mother found her with a bottles worth spread in front of her on the floor. She thinks that her daughter ingested at least one, possibly more. We contact poison control for recommendations. We then lavage her (pump her stomach), and squirt in some activated charcoal. This is really just pure stupidity on the part of parents. People are always leaving potentially toxic compounds out where toddlers can get to them. We admit this child even though she would have likely done fine regardless. That one in a million chance of bad outcome could cost you dearly if it were to come through.

Fourth is a 25-day-old white male with some nasal congestion. This is little more than a well baby check. Here is another common story. This is a first child. True to form, parents of a first child spaz out about every little thing.

Fifth is a 34-year-old white male with a two month history of oral thrush (a fungus infection with Candida albicans that produces painful friable white patches in the mouth). Surprisingly he has a doctor, but he hasn't contacted him. This guy's symptoms are no better or worse today, but somehow it's an emergency today. I put him on some Nystatin (an antifungal) and strongly suggest that he follow-up.

The real issue though is why a 34-year-old male with no other medical problems has oral thrush. It makes you start thinking about things like AIDS, or other immune compromising disorders.

Sixth is a 92-year-old white male from the nursing home with a decreased level of consciousness. He looks to be knocking on death's door and is not real long for the world. The patient and his family just want comfort measures which begs the question of why was he brought to the Emergency Department? He's had a recent pneumonia, and just wants to exit the world comfortably. I talk it over with his family and his doctor, and we sent him back to the Nursing Home to (ultimately) die a (hopefully) easy death.

In the middle of this we've also got a 97-year-old demented white female, also from the nursing home, with one day of low abdominal pain. She's got a good urinary tract infection going on. There's also a sclerotic lesion in a vertebra, but that's really a moot point. Who's going to aggressively diagnose and treat a demented 97-year-old with a bone lesion? I mention the findings to her regular doctor, and send her back to the nursing home on an antibiotic and an analgesic.

Then to complete our laceration three-fer, I see a 75-year-old white male who cut his left index finger with a knife. It takes three sutures and is back together. It's pretty boring.

Oh joy, I get a 51-year-old white male who had a ladder fall on his head at home. Of course he works at UNEM and sees doctor NONE. He has a superficial laceration, which is hardly more than a scratch. And then we get to the real agenda…He wants some Tylenol with codeine. He says his dentist gives them to him, and that he's run out. Of course here in the ER we practice McMedicine, and you know our motto, "Have it your way…" Fine, I gave him a few Tylenol with codeine.

6:00 PM

Now here's a real emergency. Its a 7-year-old white female with recurring head lice. She had been tried with RID, but they're back. The mother didn't bother to contact their regular doctor, but brought her to my Emergency Department instead. Whatever…I put her on NIX and send her on her way.

Then we have a 86-year-old white female who had a ground level fall at home. She complains of right hip, low back, and bilateral knee pain. All of her X-rays are fine and she is weight bearing. This can be treated symptomatically, with follow-up as needed.

There's also a 3-year-old white male who ran into a door and managed a right eyebrow laceration. It's very superficial, and really doesn't need anything. The mom gets wound instructions, a head sheet, and is sent along.

More orthopedics, a 12-year-old white male who jammed his right small finger at football practice. He's split the end of one of the bones in that finger. He's splinted and follow-up is arranged.

Then one of my favorites, a 26-year-old white female who was in a minor car wreck three weeks ago and is having increasing back pain. Of course it's a crisis on a Friday night. Everything is normal in my evaluation. She is put on my routine back pain regimen.

Next is an unusual one, a 28-year-old white male who was stung on the tongue by a honeybee that was in his drinking cup. He's supposedly got an allergy to bees. There's been no reaction so far. He's given some Decadron (a steroid) and Vistaril (an antihistamine) and watched. He has no reaction and is released with recommendations.

Then I see a 17-year-old white male was struck on the top of the head playing football. He has no recollection of the event. He's also got neck pain and tingling in his hands and feet. He gets a head scan and neck scan. They're both normal, and his symptoms resolve spontaneously. He's likely got a mild concussion and neck sprain. He's released with head injury instructions. This qualifies as a grade III concussion, so he's out of the game for at least a couple of weeks.

From the same group I get a 17-year-old white male who took a helmet blow to the left hip and thigh. He acts like he's dying. Everything is normal, and he is just bruised. You'd think if these kids were going to be doing these foolish and potentially dangerous sports they'd be made of sterner stuff.

There's been a tuberculosis scare at the local shelter. An 18-year-old and two 26-year-olds come in wanting to be tested for TB. I am aware of the alleged exposure. I contact the health department and determine that it poses no risk to these folks. They are advised and referred to the local health clinic where TB tests can be done if they want to pursue it.

Next is a 26-year-old white female who has had several hours of nausea, vomiting, and diarrhea. She's very dramatic. When I was a kid, we'd call this the stomach flu, we'd drink 7-up, and stay close to the bathroom. Oh how times have changed. I give her some IV fluids and antiemetics. She's feeling all-better. Isn't that special. She gets routine stomach flu instructions, symptomatic medicines, and is sent on her way.

Then I get a 60-year-old white male who comes in with one hour of chest pain. He's well over 300 pounds and has every known cardiac risk factor known to man. He's already had a bypass and multiple angioplasties. His last angioplasty was just a couple of weeks ago. His EKG is nonspecific and his cardiac enzymes are negative. He is rapidly rendered pain free with nitrates. He's a keeper and is whisked upstairs.

Next there's a 12-year-old white male who had his left wrist over extended while playing football. On X-ray he's busted his wrist, but it's in good alignment. It is splinted and follow-up arranged.

Lastly, there's a 12-year-old white male. He and his buddy were shooting one another with BB guns. He took a round in the chest that broke the skin. It's little more than a scratch. No BB is left in him. He's chastised severely and sent on his way.

Stupid, stupid, stupid…But it's definitely the type of thing a 12-year-old does.

I have a brief reprieve where I'm able to finish my dictations. Then shift change hits, and I am out of here…

12:00 AM

Shift 15
"All good things come to an end, and no good deed goes unpunished."

Sunday—18 Hours

12:00 PM

Well we're off and running.

I've had a 50-year-old white male passed off to me with upper abdominal pain. He has a history of pancreatitis (an inflammation of the pancreas). His lab is pending, but it looks and smells like flare of his pancreatitis again. He's already had 10 milligrams of IV Morphine (a strong narcotic pain medicine) with little improvement.

I've also got a 49-year-old white female with low back pain. She thinks she has a kidney infection. It's been going on for about a week. Her urinalysis is normal, as is her exam. She doesn't want to entertain that this could be musculoskeletal, despite the reproducible tenderness she has over the muscle groups in her back. She does agree to treat it with Advil for a while and see if it improves.

Hot off the press. Our abdominal pain patient's amylase and lipase (these are pancreatic enzymes measurable in blood) are through the roof. It's completely consistent with acute pancreatitis. He says he hasn't been drinking in the last 6 months, but does have quite a prior drinking history. I'm betting he's been off the wagon, but who knows and who cares. It doesn't change what we do. Well he'll be admitted and out of my hair in short order.

We've also got a 76-year-old white female with upper abdominal and low mid chest pain. Within the last week she's had a significant work-up for these symptoms. She's had a normal stress test, normal lab, and a normal Upper GI (an X-ray test where a person drinks some barium). The pain is worse after eating certain foods and also worse when lying down. She has known GERD (gastroesophageal reflux) as well as a history of esophageal stricture that has required dilation. I'm betting that this is where her pain is coming from. She also comments on episodes of right upper abdominal pain radiating to the back that also occurs after eating. So her gall bladder is also a possibility. We'll check it all, but I'm not confident we'll find anything.

There's also a 61-year-old white female with pain and burning with urination as well as blood in her urine. Her urine does look pretty nasty. We'll see what the urinalysis shows.

I've also got a 44-year-old white male contact wearer with two days of increasing right eye redness, drainage, and pain. He has a small corneal abrasion on dye exam. We give him some Tobrex (an antibiotic eye drop) and some pain medicine. He needs to leave his contacts out till things resolve.

The 61-year-old with painful urination has a really junky urinalysis, but this is no big surprise. She just needs an antibiotic. I'll put her on Bactrim (a sulfa antibiotic) for a week. She'll be fine.

Surprise, surprise, our 76-year-old white female with the chest and abdominal pain gets a Cadillac work-up without really finding much. I even did an abdominal ultrasound that was pretty much normal. When I talked to her further, I did hit on how the symptoms were much worse after ice cream but not affected by McDonald ice cream. Well McDonald ice cream is not made with milk products, but is a palm oil derivative. This patient likely has lactose intolerance in addition to her reflux and esophageal stricture. We'll have her stop eating milk products for a few days and see if it helps. We'll also increase her Prevacid (a proton pump inhibitor that reduces stomach acid production), in case her reflux is contributing to her symptoms. She can follow-up with her regular doctor.

Oh Joy, an overdose. It's a real ditz. This is an 18-year-old white female who allegedly took 50 extra strength Tylenol and a similar number of Excedrin about 12 hours prior to presentation. She's brought in by her family, and isn't talking much. After twelve hours there's really not a lot to do except check levels. If she's really taken this amount of Tylenol, then she could be dead in a couple of days from liver failure. I'm skeptical though. Excedrin has caffeine and aspirin in it. This amount should have her caffeine toxic with her heart racing to beat the band. The aspirin should have her very acidotic. I would expect her to be breathing very fast to compensate for the acidosis the aspirin would produce, or for her to be near comatose. She's neither, so you really have to wonder how much of what she's actually taken. The nurse calls the local police to get an emergency committal. Even if she's taken nothing, she's obviously a potential risk to herself and needs a psychiatric evaluation whether she wants one or not.

Meanwhile, I see a 34-year-old white male. He was a restrained driver in a motor vehicle accident. His car was rear-ended, but there was little damage to the car. There was no loss of consciousness. He complains of left face, left shoulder and diffuse neck pain. His exam is benign, so he's sent off for some medico-legal X-rays. They're all normal, although there's quit a bit of degenerative change for someone so young. He's just got a bit of neck sprain and seatbelt contusion. This is treated symptomatically.

This is followed by a 21-year-old Hispanic male who's had burning with urination for a month. This is another doctor NONE patient whose decided it's a crisis today. His urinalysis is weakly positive, but this is more likely a sexually transmitted disease. I swab him and treat him both for sexually transmitted disease as well as for a urinary tract infection. He'll need follow-up, especially if he's got chlamydia or the like.

With our overdose, she tells the police that she had only taken perhaps 15 Tylenol. We get her levels back and they're more consistent with this. This is a harmless amount for this patient. She now admits that she was trying to hurt herself, and recognizes that she needs help. I coordinate with the local psychiatric facility that takes these folks, and get her on the way.

We get so many of these suicide attempts where folks make a half-hearted effort. We often joke that we need to provide an instruction manual so they get it right. Most of these folks aren't really trying to get the job done. Hell, many times they take the pills and then immediately call 911. Often it seems they're trying to get attention from family or significant others. Folks who really want to kill themselves tend to get the job done. They do definitive things. True, they occasionally botch it. For example, if they try and remove their head with a shotgun, but just manage to blow off their face. Ah, well…

I see a 9-day-old white male with a red draining left eye. The child was born by C-section, so this is likely a routine conjunctivitis. I put him on some antibiotic eye drops and recommend follow-up.

Boy we are just off to the races. People keep coming in.

First is a 6-year-old white male who was doing foolish things with his bike. He fell and lacerated his upper gums. Of course he was wearing no protective gear. He has no other specific complaints. I filmed his face to ensure there were no facial fractures. The gum laceration is more of an abrasion and needs no specific treatment. It'll heal in a few days.

Second, I've got a 24-year-old white male who jabbed his left hand with a screwdriver. It just needs to be cleaned and a single suture.

I also see a 17-month-old white male with cough and wheezing. He's got a history of asthma, and had just finished a course of Augmentin (an antibiotic) for bronchitis. His oxygenation is fine and his chest X-ray is normal. This just seems to be some exacerbation of his asthma. I put him on some Prelone (a steroid), and will increase his nebulizer treatments. He needs to be rechecked later in the week.

Fourth, I see a 15-year-old diabetic female with sore throat, cough, and congestion. She's already on an antibiotic. Her mother wanted her checked for strep. We do a quick strep test that is, of course, negative. The antibiotic that she is on is adequate for a strep infection. She's got a little viral illness, and can to treat this symptomatically. Of course she also needs to watch her blood sugars a bit more closely. They can be more labile any time a diabetic gets an illness.

Fifth, is one of our frequent visitors. It's a 51-year-old, morbidly obese, white female with two weeks of back pain. She's in frequently with this complaint. If she were to loose 200 pounds, her problem would likely go away. It has been a while since her back had been filmed so I did this tonight. It has a lot of degenerative change, the product of years of abuse, but is otherwise fine. I gave her my standard back sprain program, and she left feeling quite a bit better.

Sixth, is a 20-year-old white male with a deformed left long finger. It was caught up in a ski rope. On the film it's just dislocated. It just needs some mild traction, and it's back to normal. I splint it for a couple of weeks to insure he regains the integrity of the joint, but it should do fine.

Seventh, I see a 3-year-old white male who had fallen at home and scraped his left elbow. When his parents checked his elbow, they noted a swollen red lesion on his forearm. Of course they are sure it is a "spider bite." It's likely just an allergic reaction to a mosquito bite, but it could be a local cellulitis, so I covered him with an antibiotic. He'll do fine.

Public awareness programs are such two edged swords. Several months ago there was a lot of publicity about the Brown Recluse spider. This is a spider that is not endemic to these parts. it can cause a nasty skin ulcer. The key television programs were even commenting that the spider isn't really seen locally. However, since that time, we've gotten huge numbers of folks who come in with mosquito bites that are sure they have Brown

Recluse bites. Ah well, it's just the nature of the business that we get the panicked worried well.

Back to the fray, eighth is an 84-year-old white female who lost her balance in the nursing home and fell. She struck the back of her head, did not lose consciousness, and has been fine since. Her local doctor had her sent over to get a head scan. The rational was that she needed it because she was on Coumadin (a blood thinner), and is thus at risk for an intracranial bleed. It seems to be a weak rationale, but we spend a thousand dollars for a normal head scan just the same.

I also see a 85-year-old white female with two days of dizziness. She had been started on Neurontin (a seizure medicine also used as a pain modifier) just the day before. She had called the on-call doctor the day before who had told her that it was likely that her symptoms were due to the Neurontin. He had her stop it and told her the symptoms should be better within 24 hours. Well now it's 24 hours later and she still feels dizzy. Of course she didn't call the doctor back but came right in. She also has a history of recurrent dizziness going back for years. Likely as not it wasn't the Neurontin that produced her symptoms, but was her recurrent vertigo. I gave her some Antivert (a dizziness medicine) and she is all-better. She can follow-up later.

Then I see a 14-year-old black male with 3 days of mid-chest pain and shortness of breath. He allegedly has a history of asthma. His chest X-ray and his peak flows are normal. He says he feels better after a treatment. I decide to treat him as exacerbation of asthma with some prednisone (a steroid) and an inhaler. I really question whether he really is an asthmatic, but even placebo effect should make him feel better.

Next is a 4-year-old white female with a fever and a frontal headache. Of course she'd not been given anything for either. Her exam was normal. We do some basic lab that was normal. She is cured with a single dose of Motrin. She's likely got a virus if anything. Ah, the wonder of Motrin. They should make that nonprescription. Oh, but wait, it is already. I guess people just haven't heard of it before.

Then we have another frequent flyer. It's a 35-year-old white female with a "migraine headache" for a week. She's been in just yesterday and had gotten everything but the kitchen sink. It really seems like all of the headache patients we see have huge psychiatric components, and this is no exception. Of course her exam is normal. I give her a full range of headache stuff: Nubain, Phenergan, DHE, Thorazine, Ativan, and she goes away.

Oh joy, more fun, a 17-year-old white female, a runaway, who's been on the streets for the last three days. She is brought in by her guardians, and they want a drug screen on her. Surprise, she tests positive for pretty much everything. Of course she denies that she's had anything. There's not a whole lot that I have to offer. She needs referral for counseling. They can see her regular doctor for that.

Then I see a 48-year-old white female with a day of right sided neck pain. She has a history of fibromyalgia and migraine headache, and has had a lot of problems with these over the last week. She thinks she feels enlarged lymph nodes in her neck, but in reality her pain is in a location where there are no lymph nodes. There's just some muscle spasm that she's feeling. She has a neck sprain with muscle spasm. This is probably related to exacerbation of the pain syndromes she has. Once I identify this to her, surprisingly she doesn't want anything more for it. She tells me she'll use the medicines she already has at home. That's a novelty.

7:00 PM

Next I see a 51-year-old white male with two days of right shoulder pain. This is worse with a deep breath. It's just below his scapula. Of course it didn't occur to him to try anything for this: Motrin, Aleve, etc. I do a chest X-ray for good measure that is normal. It can be treated symptomatically. He's likely pulled something.

This is followed by a 47-year-old white female who fell this morning. She complains of left lower leg pain. She does have some minimal bruising about her little toe. I film everything, and they're all normal. This also can be treated symptomatically.

Then there's a 4-year-old white male with a fever and sore throat for 3 days. His strep test is negative, but he does have an ear infection in his right ear. The mother does say then, that he has been pulling at that ear. I put him on an antibiotic, and he should do fine.

Next is a 12-month-old white female who has had cold symptoms and been fussy today. The mother called the nurse line to see what dose of Pediacare (an over the counter cold medicine) to use, and was told to come to the Emergency Room and have the child checked. I can't really understand this. The child has a cold. I gave the mother the appropriate dose (1 and a half droppers) and send her on her way.

Sometimes you just have to shake your head. Next is a 61-year-old white female who was riding a new bike she had just purchased, and fell off. She's complaining of left shoulder pain. Surprise, she's managed to break her proximal humerus (the bone in the upper arm) just below the shoulder. This is treated with a shoulder immobilizer and follow-up. She's not going to be riding her bike for a couple months.

Then I've got a 29-year-old white female with two weeks of sinus drainage, cough and the like. She is on just about every medicine known to man. Now she's got decreased hearing in her left ear. The eardrum looks fine, it's just that it's bulging out towards me. She likely got some Eustachian tube dysfunction (the tubes exiting in the back of the throat that equalize the pressure behind the ear drums) due to her viral illness. She's upset that I don't have any way to immediately cure her.

Next I see another of our frequent visitors. This is a 71-year-old white male who really belongs in a nursing home. He's complaining of pain from his mouth to his penis. He had a tooth extracted a couple days ago and is having pain from that site. His other pain complaints are long-standing, of years duration, and unchanged. The extraction site looks fine, so I put him on an antibiotic for good measure and give him some

Vicodin (a mild narcotic pain medicine). He can follow-up with his dentist in the morning.

There's a 12-year-old white male who was fighting with his brother and put his right arm through a window. He's got a nice laceration of his forearm. It's not seriously injured, but it does take a two layered closure. He gets 13 sutures and is out of here.

Then we have another very common problem. It's a 48-year-old white female with uncontrolled diabetes, and end stage complications. She's had increasing redness and swelling of her right foot for almost a week. She's also had infection in the bones of that foot that required toe amputation. You'd think she would pay closer attention, but oh no. The lab and X-ray suggests that she may have a new bone infection. Given her history she needs admission for IV antibiotics and surgery evaluation.

Okay, next is a 26-year-old white female with right upper wisdom tooth pain as well as some sinus symptoms. The tooth is partially erupted and the area looks infected. I cover her with an antibiotic and give her some pain medicine. I impress on her that she needs to see a dentist or oral surgeon. Those wisdom teeth need to come out.

Next is a 19-year-old white female who feels "shaky." She had some heat exhaustion yesterday after a Soccer game and had gotten a couple of liters of fluid in another ER. There's nothing to suggest that this is going on today. She seems to be having a panic attack, and does state that she has been under a lot of stress. She's cured with some vitamin "X," Xanax (a tranquilizer).

Then I see a 17-year-old white female who stepped on a piece of glass and lacerated her foot. She's drunk as a skunk, and refuses to have it sutured. We clean it up, and send her on her way.

12:00 AM

The Witching hour and, our 23-year-old white female with the chronic headache returns. She wants to be admitted. I guess she has been harassing the local on-call doctor all evening. I give him a call. He caves and admits her.

Next is a 52-year-old white male with 1 month of left sided flank pain and blood in the urine. He does have a history of kidney stones. At no time in the last month has he had it investigated, and it's a crisis tonight. It's not any better or worse than it has been all along. He does have blood in his urine, and so I do an IVP. It's normal. I'll treat him for a pyelonephritis (a bladder infection that has ascended to the kidneys), and he can follow-up with the local urologist at his convenience.

Then we get a 62-year-old white male with difficulty swallowing for the last 8 hours. He's had recurrent problems with this for the last 15 years, but never had it looked into. Apparently this started after eating some meat. He's probably got a meat impaction. I give him some Ativan (a tranquilizer) and glucagon (a hyperglycemic agent that incidentally relaxes the esophagus) and he's cured in about an hour. He needs his esophagus visualized.

The Emergency Department is finally empty. This is the first time I've had to work on my dictations since I came on duty. I spend a couple hours getting caught up.

3:00 AM

Another crisis, a 51-year-old white female with 3 hours of diarrhea and crampy abdominal pain. Of course everything is normal. I give her some IV fluids, some Toradol, and some Compazine and she's feeling like a new woman.

Then we get an 84-year-old white female with a recent history of stroke. She's had some urinary incontinence getting up to go to the bathroom. She's brought in by her family. They are sure she's having another stroke, even though there are no localizing symptoms. A full stroke work-up is negative, and when all is said and done the family admits they may have over-reacted. The patient is already on Aspirin and Plavix (platelet active medicines that reduce clotting). We agree on some watchful waiting for now, and treat her urinary tract infection.

I also get a 41-year-old white female in by squad with sharp right sided chest pain. Everything is normal. She is pretty much cured with some Toradol (an anti-inflammatory). The next shift comes in and takes over the patient. The family is spazzing out, so the next shift decides to do a spiral CT to rule out pulmonary embolus. And this is the time for me to hit the road.

6:00 AM

I am out of here...And so ends a month in the Emergency Department.

Epilogue
"Much ado about nothing…"

As I go back and re-edit these chapters for the zillionth time, my initial thoughts and reflections are validated. This really does present a cross section of what we get in the Emergency Room in the summertime. As you can see, so much of it has no business being there. The bulk of the rest falls into a broad range of themes. This includes things like cuts, broken bones, chest pain and the like. There is the occasional excitement, but it's all in a days work. For folks that work in the field, there is little that makes them panic, or gets their heart racing. Even with Codes (cardiopulmonary arrest and the like), you go in with the understanding that the patient is already dead, and if you can bring them back, so much the better. If not, well, they're still dead.

The Emergency Department is not about drama, at least not most of the time. There isn't one amazing save after another. Similarly, there isn't one tumultuous death after another. Usually the saves are just as anticlimactic as the deaths. If you're doing your job, you don't normally let a situation deteriorate to the point where you need an amazing save, at least if you can help it. Similarly, most of the deaths are expected, and your task is really just to ease the transition.

Likewise, there aren't a lot of big ethical dilemmas. Yes, they do sometimes occur, but potential ethical problems usually fall within the scope of situations that you've already given a lot of thought to. You typically have an approach to the problem and an answer to the dilemma that you're able to live with.

Unfortunately, much of Emergency Medicine is about legal consequences. Not only is this the specialty with the most litigation exposure, but there are continually expanding legal consequences levied by State and Federal organizations under the umbrella of EMTALA, Medicare, Medicaid, and the like.

A broad cross section of people are drawn to the practice of emergency medicine. This includes its share of idealists and adrenaline junkies. After a time, though there are moments where you feel you have really accomplished something and saved a life, the majority of the time you just feel drained. It is not unexpected that emergency medicine has one of the highest burn-out rates. Seven years is the number I routinely hear tossed about, and it seems right on the money. You see the worst of everything and everyone; so it is perhaps the norm that your idealism is replaced by cynicism as it wears you down. To those of you who are considering a career in this field, I would caution you to go into it with your eyes wide open, and in full possession of the facts. I would also advise you to have a fallback plan for when you reach that point where you dread going back to work yet another shift. Emergency medicine truly has the soul of a beast, and it will devour the unprepared.

The Author
"No Doubt..." (an inside joke)

Well I guess I should say something about myself, if only because it makes such an unusual story. I grew up mostly in small towns in the Pacific Northwest in the 60's and 70's. I was a nerdy kind of guy who spent a lot of time in the library. I graduated high school early, and went to a small private college in my home state. Shortly after my seventeenth birthday, I started out working on a multiple major in Chemistry, Physics, Biology, Mathematics, and Economics.

After pursuing my ambitious multiple major for a time, I became anxious to get out of school and into the "real world". I was closest to completing a pure physics degree, and began directing my energies towards that end. It had occurred to me that I didn't know what a person could do, job wise, with a degree in physics, so I went to the chair of the physics department and asked his advice. His response in a nutshell was, "Well (pause), you could go to graduate school..."

It was shortly after this that my growing disillusionment gelled and, in the manner of the young and stupid, I dropped out of school. Unfortunately when you're nineteen, it doesn't matter how bright you are, you were pretty well unemployable back in the mid-70's.

I decided to go into the military, and enlisted in the United States Air Force. What I discovered is that slave labor is not a lot of fun. I looked to see if there were any Air Force education programs that I could get involved with in order to get back on track with my future. I wanted to get out of the enlisted ranks, and given that I still had something over three years of obligation that I still owed, a commissioning program seemed my best bet. Unfortunately I was told I didn't qualify as my last semester of college was such a shambles that it just killed my GPA. This left me in something of a quandary as to what to do next.

One thing I found I was able to do in the military was take advanced placement tests (CLEP, DANTES, ACT, and the like). These were free of charge for an Airman on active duty, and so I took them all. Over a 6-8 month period I accrued something over 100 semester hours in college credit via examination. With this, in addition to the 110 semester hours I had from College, I felt that it should be enough to get some kind of degree. I contacted several colleges, including the one I had previously attended, to see what options I had available. I was told invariably that I had to complete the last 36 odd semester hours on-campus. "Really stupid", I thought. I knew there had to be a better way.

I combed the nation for a college that catered to non-traditional students and found two. Both acted as credit banks to put together college credit from other institutions. I applied to both simultaneously. The one that responded quickest required that I complete additional 12 semester hours of senior level coursework or above. The other took forever to reply.

I enrolled as an unclassified student in a graduate program in Health Sciences that was available on the Air Force base where I was stationed. I completed the required work in about 5 months. In the end, I graduated with a Bachelor of Science in General Studies, and applied to OTS (Officer Training School).

Simultaneously with my OTS application, I applied for training in the fields of Missile Maintenance or Space Systems. I had grown up during the space race, had dreamed of being an astronaut, and felt that this would be a path close to that aspiration. I was told that because I had had calculus in college that I was instead going to be a Communications Electronics Officer. It seems they don't get many folks who've completed calculus.

I spent 4 months in Officer Training School and was commissioned a Second Lieutenant in the Air Force at the age of twenty-one. I then spent 8 months in Communications Electronics School, plus an additional 4 months in Communication Computer School.

Throughout my time in the military, I never really did anything that required calculus. This must have something to do with the classic oxymoron about military intelligence, but it's hard to say.

I spent a total of 7 years in the military playing computer geek, before leaving to seek my fortune at the age of twenty-seven. During that time, the Air Force spent a tremendous amount for me to attend a wide range of military and commercial schools. I have estimated that I spent 3-4 years of my military stint in one school or another.

Towards the end of my time in the military I became interested in construction, and founded a construction company. A partner and I built houses in our spare time for about three years. This was a poor time for the construction industry. We worked a lot, but didn't make much for our efforts. It was an interesting experience, but perhaps not the best use of my time.

After the military, I went to work as a computer consultant for a DOD contractor. I did this for about 5 years. This was my transition from military computer geek to corporate computer geek.

Way back in High School I had thought of going into Medicine. This thought had recurred during the time that I was taking the graduate courses in health sciences before my commissioning. I had talked about possibly going to Medical School all along the way, but hadn't taken any definitive steps.

At twenty-eight, I found myself single and unattached. I had spent the better part of ten years talking about how I wanted to go to Medical School, and I felt I needed to either get on with it or forget it.

I spent two years repeating the pre-medicine basics while getting my financial house in order. I applied to the local medical school, and surprisingly to me, I was accepted immediately.

I spent the next four years in medical school, and managed to graduate with distinction. I was actually interested in Pathology as a path to genetics research (This was something I developed an interest in along the way. I see it as the future of medicine, but that's another story entirely). Unfortunately, there was an untimely surplus of folks wanting to be Pathologists, and so I wound up in my first fallback position, internal medicine (adult medicine).

While I was in my residency I moonlighted in several Emergency Departments around the area, and found that I liked it better than internal medicine. (Actually it was a bit more than JUST moonlighting. I was working so many hours at so many Emergency Departments, that I was making more than most of the staff physicians in my internal medicine training program.) It is noteworthy that the vast majority of emergencies in an Emergency Department are adult medical emergencies, and so internal medicine was not such a bad match.

There were no emergency medicine residencies locally available, and so I arranged for additional training in pediatrics, obstetrics, and the like to round out my formal adult medicine training. I completed my (enhanced) internal medicine residency, and have worked exclusively in emergency medicine since. To date I've worked almost exactly five years in the field.

Since residency, I have spent a year and a half of my spare time building a house (a flashback to my construction days) for my family. I then spent another year and a half completing a MBA (This was motivated both by an interest in investing to obtain financial independence, as well as in anticipation of perhaps founding a biotechnology company down the road). Through this I've maintained an interest in genetics and gene therapy, and will start a formal Ph.D. program in molecular biology and molecular genetics in about a year from the date of this writing. I will likely leave clinical medicine at that time, hopefully in advance of that 7-year burnout period I mentioned earlier.

24574330R00104

Made in the USA
Lexington, KY
23 July 2013